AF271503

Tanya L. Fernandez, MS, PA-C, IBCLC, is an assistant professor at the University of Colorado Child Health Associate/Physician Assistant (CHA/PA) Program. She is a board-certified physician assistant and lactation consultant who has spent her clinical career working with families, children, and adolescents in underserved and high-risk populations. She joined the faculty at the CHA/PA Program in 2016 and holds both didactic and clinical education responsibilities within the program. She is the coauthor of *The Physician Assistant Student's Guide to the Clinical Year: Pediatrics*.

For PAs, NPs, and Other Healthcare Providers

Tanya L. Fernandez, MS, PA-C, IBCLC

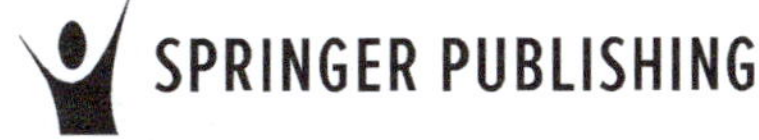

Springer Publishing Company, LLC
11 West 42nd Street, New York, NY 10036
www.springerpub.com
connect.springerpub.com/

Acquisitions Editor: Suzanne Toppy
Compositor: diacriTech

ISBN: 978-0-8261-5646-4
ebook ISBN: 978-0-8261-5647-1
DOI: 10.1891/9780826156471

24 25 / 5 4 3

The author and the publisher of this Work have made every effort to use sources believed to be reliable to provide information that is accurate and compatible with the standards generally accepted at the time of publication. Because medical science is continually advancing, our knowledge base continues to expand. Therefore, as new information becomes available, changes in procedures become necessary. We recommend that the reader always consult current research and specific institutional policies before performing any clinical procedure or delivering any medication. The author and publisher shall not be liable for any special, consequential, or exemplary damages resulting, in whole or in part, from the readers' use of, or reliance on, the information contained in this book. The publisher has no responsibility for the persistence or accuracy of URLs for external or third-party Internet websites referred to in this publication and does not guarantee that any content on such websites is, or will remain, accurate or appropriate.

Library of Congress Cataloging-in-Publication Data
Library of Congress Control Number: 2021906487

Tanya L. Fernandez: https://orcid.org/0000-0003-2618-4605

Contact sales@springerpub.com to receive discount rates on bulk purchases.

Publisher's Note: **New and used products purchased from third-party sellers are not guaranteed for quality, authenticity, or access to any included digital components.**

Printed in the United States of America by Gasch Printing.

Dedicated to those with whom I share our great nest. My wonderful husband and my two beautiful children have brought the NEST & FLY concepts to my life. You helped me navigate the uncertainty of writing this book, and you nourished me with your undying support, love, and frequent delivery pizza. You encouraged me to exercise my imagination, reminded me to sleep, and pushed me forward on my current trajectory.

To my moms, you are the nest from which I have been able to fly. Thank you for letting me stand on the edge of the nest and eventually pushing me off, knowing I had my wings to fly.

CONTENTS

Amy Akerman, MPAS, PA-C, Assistant Professor, University of Colorado Child Health Associate/ Physician Assistant Program, Aurora, Colorado

Wesley Gallegos, MPAS, CHA/PA-C, Instructor of Pediatrics, Child Health Clinic, Children's Hospital Colorado, Aurora, Colorado

Laura Swanson, RN, MSN, CPNP, Pediatric Nurse Practitioner, Adjoint Faculty, University of Colorado School of Nursing, Aurora, Colorado

Many parents know to seek healthcare when their children are sick, but well-child visits are equally important when it comes to keeping children healthy. During the well-child visit, clinicians can focus on parental concerns such as sleeping and eating and on preventive factors that help keep children healthy, such as immunizations, nutrition, and development. Advanced practice providers (APPs) play a pivotal role caring for children and families across the pediatric continuum from infancy through young adulthood. A quick-access resource, such as the *Well-Child Primary Care Pocket Guide*, will help APPs and other healthcare providers responsible for the primary care of children stay current with the latest recommendations for pediatric well-child care.

The *Well-Child Primary Care Pocket Guide* was written by an experienced pediatric clinician and provides current and clinically relevant information for healthcare providers working with pediatric patients. A stand-out feature of the *Well-Child Primary Care Pocket Guide* is that it is the only pocket-sized resource that guides you through pediatric well visits using a unique, logical, and easy-to-remember mnemonic: NEST & FLY. This mnemonic facilitates understanding of concepts related to well-child care such as nutrition, elimination, and sleep.

The *Well-Child Primary Care Pocket Guide* is an excellent resource for both novice and experienced clinicians. Throughout this guide, you will find useful information that can be immediately applied to clinical practice. The chapters are organized to be consistent with the AAP schedule of well-child visits. This structure will help to ensure that in each well-child visit you gather age-relevant information about important factors such as nutrition, sleep, elimination, and activity/development.

The *Well-Child Primary Care Pocket Guide* contains a variety of features that sets it apart from other pediatric books. It is presented in a practical and easily understandable bullet-point format. This pocket guide is uniquely designed with easy-to-navigate, color-coded tables to help clinicians quickly locate information needed to assess the pediatric patient's nutrition, elimination, and development. This *Pocket Guide* also provides you with key interviewing strategies and questions to gather an updated history, as well as step-by-step guidelines for the head-to-toe physical examination.

The *Well-Child Primary Care Pocket Guide* is portable and well-organized and contains entries that can be quickly accessed. These features make it easy to use in busy clinical settings. Overall, the unique format and comprehensive information provided in the *Well-Child Primary Care Pocket Guide* makes it an excellent resource for healthcare providers working with pediatric patients. It will be an asset to your practice whether you are providing well-child care as a new clinician or a seasoned professional.

Mikki Meadows-Oliver, PhD, PNP-BC, FAAN
Clinical Professor
New York University School of Nursing

In the P. D. Eastman early reader classic *Are You My Mother?*, the baby bird hatches into his perfectly crafted, but empty, nest. In an effort to find his mother, he drops to the ground not yet able to fly, without a plan to find her or even an idea of what he is looking for. He, nonetheless, seeks to find her, wandering through an overwhelming world asking hit-or-miss queries of the characters he comes across.

For many, the pediatric health maintenance visit can parallel the hatchling's adventures. It is necessary and important to do, but because of the dramatic developmental and psychosocial changes that occur from birth through adolescence, keeping track of the ever-changing recommendations and the various components of the well visit can feel overwhelming and aimless without an organized approach. This book provides a standardized and organized framework for conducting the well visit. My unique NEST & FLY memory tools (i.e., NEST: **n**utrition, **e**limination/exercise, **s**leep, **t**racking; FLY: **f**amily support, **l**earned skills, **y**our tools) are carried through the guide for a consistent presentation of key information about the well-child visit for children ages newborn to 18 years. In an easy-to-use, tabular format, this pocket guide will help busy physician assistants, nurse practitioners, or other health professionals working with children quickly identify questions to ask and the current recommendations for each age group. As a grab-and-go guide, the tables are organized into the important well-visit components, such as age appropriate:

- Nutrition and exercise recommendations
- Elimination variations and struggles
- Sleep patterns, evolving sleep issues, and current recommendations to support healthy development
- Expected changes in growth parameters
- Family/community supports and potential barriers to consider discussing during the visit
- Developmental milestones to monitor
- Physical exam components and possible normal variants seen at different ages
- Age-specific screenings and immunizations
- Anticipatory guidance talking points

This book is designed to be a pocket resource for busy clinicians without the bulk and detail of a textbook. In developing this book, I pulled from the suggestions from learners in an academic pediatric practice, both advanced practice providers and residents, and incorporated the components that practicing providers with decades of experience noted to be important. This blend of rookie and seasoned practitioner feedback has created a book that is easy to use and gives quick practical guidance. Whether you are an experienced physician assistant, a newly minted nurse practitioner, a professional working with children, or a health professions student in your pediatric internship, this book will serve you well both in and out of the exam room.

Organized by age, color-coded tables are divided into newborns and infants, toddlers and preschoolers, school-aged children, and tweens and teens. Each age group has four all-in-one, quick glance tables with an overview of everything you need at your fingertips.

As you perform your interview, you will have some guiding principles to help you simultaneously collect a thorough history while also providing counseling and education when necessary.

I'd like to thank the peer reviewers who took time away from their primary jobs and their patients to ensure that this book was of the highest quality and of the greatest utility to primary care providers. Your suggestions and insight were invaluable, and I am so honored to have worked with each of you.

Thank you to my editor, Suzanne Czehut Toppy, for getting behind the idea of this book and believing that it was a worthwhile project. I appreciate your guidance and expertise throughout this process.

Organized by age groups and the specific well visits within that age group, you'll find information on newborns and infants, toddlers and preschoolers, school-aged children, and tweens and teens synthesized in color-coded tables for easy reference.

This guide can be used to prepare for a specific aged visit by flipping to the corresponding age and reviewing the nutritional recommendations, elimination or exercise routines, sleep patterns, and developmental milestones. As you perform your interview, you will have some guiding principles to help you simultaneously collect a thorough history while also provide counseling and education when necessary.

You can also use this pocket guide in the exam room to jumpstart the interview, open up discussion, and navigate some of the more sensitive topics or questions. Many of these questions may be interchangeable from one age group to the next, so, when appropriate, feel free to mix and match ideas for questions from different ages to best meet your patient's needs.

Finally, this pocket guide provides an introduction to the novel NEST & FLY mnemonic approach to well visits. Short vignettes that capture the ABCs of the ages and stages of pediatric development from newborn to 18 years old are combined with information on the needed screenings, immunizations, and documentation for an appropriately thorough well visit.

The pediatric well visit, often referred to as the well-child check (WCC), is a visit scheduled specifically to assess a pediatric patient's overall physical health, update the health history, assess growth trajectories, and gauge development. These visits are also a time to address issues related to preventive care, answer parent or patient questions, and understand the family's social situation. The majority of the visit focuses on gathering age-appropriate information, evaluating the family or patient's response to the current age or stage, examining the patient, and providing anticipatory guidance and other preventive health measures.

NEST & FLY: TAKING THE HISTORY

When a healthy child presents for a routine well-child care visit, a systematic way of capturing the important information about a child's growth and development is very helpful, especially given the nuanced differences in the ages and stages of pediatrics. One way to think about these visits is through an analogy to baby birds. Birds create a nest that is just the right size, shape, and depth to protect their hatchlings. In that **NEST**, they feed (*Nutrition*) and care for the babies (think changing diapers and *Elimination* or tummy time and *Exercise*), *Sleep* with the chicks, and *Track* the chicks' growth and health. Chicks are allowed to **FLY** once they are developmentally ready for this task. Flying requires *Family* support, *Learned* skills (developmental milestones), and the *Young* one's tools to put it all together or in this case *Your* tools.

Growth can be influenced by nutrition and seen in patterns of elimination. Growth is greatly influenced by sufficient sleep, and should be tracked over time. On the other hand, development is supported by family interactions and is driven by learning that can be measured by your tools.

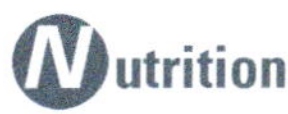

Nutrition

Determining the appropriate nutritional status of a pediatric patient will allow you to assess for potential deficiencies and provide guidance for patients and parents on changing demands and needs. However, nutrition is more than feeding frequency and portion sizes. To identify the important concepts under nutrition, **NaVIGATeD** is a useful acronym.

Asking families and patients about the types and quantities of **Na**tural foods (fruits, vegetables, and protein sources) can quickly determine whether the child may be at risk for **V**itamin deficiencies. Understanding vitamin supplementation recommendations is also important. **I**ron sources are an important component of the nutrition history throughout the pediatric spectrum because anemia can contribute to poor growth and developmental delays. The amount of whole **G**rains and **A**dded sugar and salt are great talking points with childhood obesity on the rise. **Te**eth and gum care are fundamental to optimal health. **D**airy is an often-forgotten dietary component.

This book is a compilation of some general recommendations for various age groups around fruit, vegetable, protein (many times also serving as the iron sources), carbohydrate, dairy, and vitamin intake. However, you should always tailor your information to the child's individual, medical, and social situation, a family's cultural preferences, and keep in mind that socioeconomic factors contribute greatly to a child's nutritional status. For patients who struggle with food insecurity, asking about government assistance use, school breakfast and lunch programs, and providing resources for food banks, summer lunch programs, backpack programs, and how to apply for assistance can be life changing.

With an increasing epidemic of childhood obesity, nutritional education and evaluation are critical for the prevention and curtailing of increasing waist sizes in pediatric patients. Understanding and sharing information on appropriate portion and serving sizes, daily requirements, and barriers to healthy eating are vital for pediatric practitioners to understand. As these requirements change with varying energy demands throughout childhood, the advice that is given to families at various ages may be dramatically different and may need to be tailored to cultural, socioeconomic, and individual activity levels.

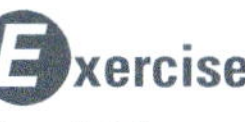limination

Elimination is a top parental observation during the early years, as parents are immersed in diaper changes and potty training. Understanding what is normal in regard to elimination and being able to provide reassurance and anticipatory guidance to families will serve you well in your family education. Elimination, both urination and defecation, is also a helpful indicator of health. Baseline query should include what type of elimination and how frequently that occurs, along with color and consistency.

Studies now show that perturbations in the gut microbiome can affect the body and brain from the neonatal period through adulthood. Stool and urine are external markers of internal health, so changes from baseline or abnormalities can offer clues to the etiology of a growth or development idiosyncrasy. Additionally, providing education and reassurance to patients and families in this domain is an important aspect of a well-child visit.

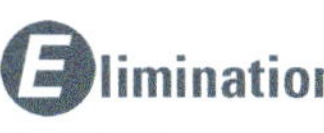xercise

As childhood obesity continues to rise despite pediatric interventions, an emphasis on physical activity and exercise should overtake much of the elimination discussion with parents after the toilet training years. Understanding normal physical activity requirements for children and adolescents, how screen time affects physical activity, and the consequences on the developing brain are critical for providing sound advice and tips and tricks to at-risk families.

Additionally, children's sports have become more and more competitive with bigger demands on pediatric bodies. Knowing appropriate limits for exercise and training can prevent overuse injuries while still encouraging early adoption of habits that may set a child up for a lifetime of physical activity.

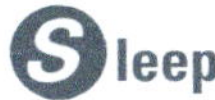

Sleep

The position during sleep, quality and quantity of sleep, routines around healthy sleep, and sleep safety are important components to consider for a screening interview. Sleep, as a topic during well visits, will change over time, but across all ages of pediatric care, the quality of sleep (for the patient or the parents), routines around sleep, and sleep safety are important to discuss. Sleep apnea and sleep disorders have become more prominent in the pediatric field, so having a working knowledge of the indicators for further testing will serve your patients and families well.

From the 1st to the 21st year of life, sleep is a common concern for parents. Parents worry that their infant isn't sleeping like other babies or that the baby sleeps too little or too long. Parents of infants are often not getting enough sleep, which can increase the risk for harm to an infant, maternal depression, or unsafe sleep practices. As children age, parents may come in with concerns about bedtime routines, struggles at bedtime, nightmares, night terrors, and nighttime awakenings. Once into the preteen and teen years, sleep cycles and sleep patterns change again, creating more questions for parents. Clearly, sleep is a big deal. Understanding the normal ranges for sleep by age, how to incorporate routines around sleep, sleep site, sleep safety, sleep position, and evidence-based sleep hygiene principles will help guide a focused discussion with a family.

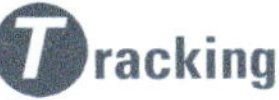

Tracking

Prior to seeing the patient, the first step in the evaluation is to review the child's growth chart, paying attention to the trajectory of previous points compared to today's point. In children younger than 2 years of age, recumbent length, weight, and HC should be plotted on a World Health Organization (WHO) growth chart. Beginning at 2, height is usually measured using a stadiometer[1-3] and can be combined with weight and age to calculate BMI. Evaluating the growth velocity and growth trends over time is more valuable than a single point on the graph, but a BMI or weight-to-length ratio can provide you with information on the proportionality of the child and may provide information on the child's nutritional status and body fat. Additionally, tracking a child's growth curves is extremely important, as a fall below the 5th percentile, moving above the 95th percentile, or crossing two major percentile lines between 2 years and puberty may indicate the child is at nutritional risk.[3,4] These changes always merit further evaluation.

Much of the tracking related to physical health comes via the vital signs. Blood pressure measurements should begin at the age of 3 and hearing and vision exams usually start at the age of 4. Beginning at 2 weeks of age, development can be tracked using serial surveillance (i.e., regular well-child exams that ask about development and monitor for red flags around development). Screening tools (standardized tools designed to identify delays by developmental domain) can be implemented as early as 2 months. Although much of the tracking done at well-child visits uses objective measures, the wise pediatric practitioner will never fail to incorporate the anecdotal observations of the family. Even without formal medical or developmental training, parents are keen observers of their children and are often the first to note a change.

Other important aspects to track are interval illness and changes in the medical, family, surgical, medication, and allergy history.

WHY IS THIS IMPORTANT?

Following growth and predictable developmental patterns can help identify a child at risk for an underlying problem earlier and allows for more therapeutic interventions. Identifying the underweight or overweight child provides opportunities to discuss nutrition, exercise, and healthy habits.

Family Situation

The family situation covers a wide expanse of topics from siblings and family structure (e.g., single-parent households, teen mother, divorced parents with shared custody, grandparents as caregivers, adoptive parents, same-sex parents, etc.) to outside resources, friends, financial stability, safety, and how the family is adjusting to a child's new age or stage. It is also the perfect place to touch on many of the psychosocial screening questions that can affect families and children, such as interpersonal or community violence, food and housing insecurity, tobacco exposure, and parental depression or coping difficulties. Using the memory tool of **FAMS** can help you remember some of the components that can affect growth or development.

- **F**amily and siblings: Asking about who lives with and cares for the child and the division of responsibilities can give you clues as to the roles that each person in the child's life may have. It also provides clues about routines and daily stressors, such as a family with a parent on military deployment, a mother who works nights, or a single-parent family. Other questions you might ask include number of siblings and ages, plans for more children, provision of childcare, and outside support such as friends, family, day-care providers, after-school care, and support groups like religious organizations or parent groups.

- **A**djustment to the age or stage: Inquiring about how the family is adjusting to the changes associated with the current developmental stage (e.g., "crying and colic") can help identify areas where families may need interventions, supports, or education. Acknowledging that each age and stage brings its own joys and challenges may allow parents or caregivers to express more fully their fears, frustrations, or disappointments. Each of these provides a springboard for further discussion, education, or even referrals for counseling.

On the other hand, hearing from the family about their adjustment and resilience may serve as an opportunity to praise the family for their successes. A great opening question when diving into this part of the FAMS tool is "What do you do best as a parent?"[5] as it allows the parent to articulate their strengths and creates an encouraging and positive environment in the exam room.

- **M**onetary concerns: The family situation would not be complete without asking about financial resources, use of government supplement programs (if applicable), insurance, and housing. Something that providers may forget is that food insecurity occurs at all levels of income, so asking families the following two key yes-or-no questions about food insecurity can help identify a family struggling with food insecurity.

  1. Within the past 12 months, did you worry about whether your food would run out before you got money to buy more?
  2. Within the past 12 months, was there ever a time when the food you bought did not last and you did not have the money to buy more?

  Affirmative answers to either of the questions would indicate that the family could benefit from additional community resources for food access.

  In addition to asking about food insecurity, screening for lower educational attainment, single-parent households headed by women, and un- or underemployment can be helpful to identify those with potential social barriers.[6]

- **S**afety: During the family aspect of the well visit, asking about interpersonal violence, marital discord, and safety can be crucial. A question as direct as "Do you feel safe in your current relationship?" or "Do you ever feel frightened by things your partner says or does?" may be enough to elicit crucial information about physical, emotional, or psychological abuse in the home.[7]

  Another aspect of ongoing safety includes the child's exposure to unsafe substances, like drugs and secondhand smoke. Although it may not be explicitly stated, asking about secondhand smoke exposure, marijuana exposure (for those states where this is legal), and vaping should be done at each visit. As the child ages, asking about these as personal exposures becomes an important aspect of the child and adolescent interview and generates helpful talking points for preventive care issues.[8] Firearms, bullying, school safety, neighborhood violence, crime, dating violence, sexual coercion, dependency, and mental health issues are all known to affect childhood development and may be areas to discuss at various well visits throughout the pediatric period.

Once families are established with a practice and a provider, much of this information is known, so it can be tempting to only address how the family is adjusting or handling a new age or stage; but periodically revisiting the psychosocial screening questions about safety, food insecurity, marital discord, and caregiver mental health is important for the overall health of the child.[5]

As children age, you may start asking the patients these questions to "break the ice" and move from low-stakes questions to more personal questions.

WHY IS THIS IMPORTANT?

Asking about the family situation provides diverse and sometimes unexpected clues about the social interactions, engagement, and social and financial environment that the child is being raised in. These elements significantly impact learning and development and can be modified in some cases with the right referrals to community resources. For adolescents, these questions can help to identify patients at higher risk for school dropout, parental discord, dating violence, and financial strain, allowing you to offer life-changing interventions.

Learning (Developmental Milestones)

The majority of pediatric well care is focused on the physical (and sexual), emotional, social, and cognitive development of infants, children, and adolescents. If you remember that development occurs in a predictable manner, starting centrally and moving peripherally or from head to toe, you may be able to predict the child's stage of development. For example, brain myelination starts in the core of the brain and moves peripherally,[9] which correlates with the overt motor development seen in early pediatrics. This is slowly supplanted by the development of language, cognitive, and social–emotional skills. Other examples of the predictable "central to peripheral" developmental progression include the following:

- Infant vision begins quite myopic and slowly improves to include peripheral and distance vision.
- The foundation of motor skills is gross motor truncal control with a slow march peripherally to fine motor control at the extremities.

- Social–emotional skills commence with a focus on understanding self and then move "peripherally" to relationships with others.
- Cognitive development begins with basic intelligence and then progresses to application of that knowledge for problem-solving.
- Communication in infants is primarily nonverbal and slowly expands to repetitive sounds, single words, two-word phrases, and short sentences by early childhood, from which the full sentences and prose of adolescence emerge.

WHY IS THIS IMPORTANT?

It is not surprising that development builds on foundational skills, which, if weak, may delay the progression of a developmental domain. Early identification and intervention for specific areas of delay or struggle is the single most influential factor in future outcomes. Additionally, offering parents anticipatory guidance around the upcoming age or stage can help them prepare and provide the most appropriate supports to ensure the greatest success.

Your Tools

Examining the growth and development of children requires a culmination of inputs to make a final diagnosis. Your interview, observation, age-appropriate physical exam, and use of screening and/or diagnostic tools all intertwine in creating a diagnosis for a child. Box 1 notes the components of a thorough well-child visit using the mnemonic NEST & FLY.

BOX 1: NEST & FLY: COMPONENTS OF A THOROUGH WELL-CHILD VISIT

NUTRITION
  NaVIGATeD
    *N*atural foods
    *V*itamins
    *I*ron sources
    *G*rains
    *A*dded sugar
    *T*eeth
    *D*airy
ELIMINATION/**E**XERCISE
  What and when?
  Consistency
SLEEP
  Position
  Quality
  Routines
  Safety/site
TRACKING

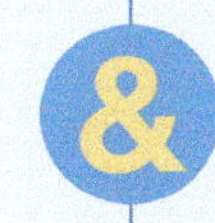

FAMILY **S**ITUATION
  Family structure, siblings, and outside support
  Adjustments to new age/stage
  Money/finances
  Safety
LEARNED **S**KILLS (**D**EVELOPMENTAL **M**ILESTONES)
  Motor (gross and fine)
  Intelligence/cognition
  Communication (verbal and nonverbal)
  Social–emotional
YOUR **T**OOLS (FOR **T**HOROUGH **A**SSESSMENT AND **P**LAN)
  Your interview with patient or family
  Your observations
  Your growth charts
  Your physical exam
  Your objective data (screenings, diagnostics)
  Your immunizations
  Your anticipatory guidance/education

PEDIATRIC AGES AND STAGES

Growth, development, and parental concerns change rapidly during infancy, childhood, and adolescence, and they can be variable within an age range. At times, it is easier to think about pediatric patients by ages, but other times it is easier to think about them as being in a particular stage or phase.

The following short vignettes will provide you with a quick glimpse at the various ages and stages seen in pediatrics.

Amazement, Anxiety, and Attachment (The Immediate Post-Partum Period)

Immediately after the birth, caregivers may have amazing or awful birth stories that can influence how easily they transition to parenthood. It is not uncommon to see parents who spend every waking moment gazing in amazement at this new addition to their lives. Often, this amazement eventually leads to some anxiety about how best to parent, the health of the newborn, and even how to afford the new family member. Attachment and bonding begins the moment the maternal hormone oxytocin begins to rise.[10] Allowing newborns to attach to the breast immediately after delivery increases further oxytocin release, beginning to solidify that bonding and those breast attachment skills.

Baby Joys, Baby Blues, and Breastfeeding (The First Month of Life)

The first month of life is a rollercoaster ride for both the newborn and the family. There are the up-and-down emotions of being giddy with joy to tearful with the baby blues, the adjustment to a new addition, and the physical, physiologic, and emotional demands of the post-partum period. Breastfeeding support for the mom–baby dyad is a primary focus at the newborn check, whereas adequate weight gain and family adjustment typically dominate the second visit of the month. Ensuring an adequate latch and addressing breastfeeding problems early, in many cases, can help normalize the struggles that many mothers face, can prevent maternal frustration and discontinuation, averts breast problems and infections, and builds an early relationship with the family that will hopefully carry forward for many more years.

A Special Note on Breastfeeding Challenges in the Early Weeks

The American Academy of Pediatrics (AAP) recommends that all infants be seen within the first week of life.[11] This is the perfect time to address feeding challenges, debunk myths, validate concerns, reinforce self-efficacy, and offer education to families regarding breastfeeding. Although newborns do instinctively find their way to the breast and latch on if unimpeded, that does not mean that it is all smooth sailing from there. The challenges associated with breastfeeding evolve throughout the postnatal period, and caregivers are not always able to articulate their fears, barriers, or concerns. Due to this inability to articulate their thoughts, it is especially important that providers create a safe space for mothers to talk about breastfeeding. Being keenly aware of what underlies some of the messages you may hear and being able to support a family with validation and education will create a more trusting and open relationship.

The top three reasons why mothers stop breastfeeding in the first month of life include the following:

- Trouble with latch and suck;
- Baby is not getting enough/not making enough milk; and
- Returning to work.[12,13]

A brief look at these and other challenges and how to approach them is included in this book in the Early and Later Breastfeeding Challenges tables, located on pages 30–33.

Contentment, Crying, and Connections (2–6 Months Old)

Once adjusted, families typically find great contentment during the first 6 months of an infant's life. They can establish some routines, sleep begins to improve, and development is overt and tangible. Physically, infants at this stage are growing rapidly, gaining chubby rolls, and double chins. Motor development quickly moves an infant from a supine, helpless position to a sitting, grasping position, and there are increasing signs of connection between the baby and her parents. However, one of the normal developmental stages that parents may not anticipate is crying. A crying infant can be very distressing for parents, so educating families at this stage about crying as a developmental milestone is essential.

Determination, Drooling, and Da-Da (9–12 Months Old)

Nine to 12 months is a time of slowed physical and gross motor development and increased social-emotional and cognitive growth. With changes in social-emotional development come an increasing autonomy, as demonstrated by self-feeding, holding toys, sitting unsupported, pulling to a stand, and maybe even taking those first few steps. Having repeated successes and autonomy often means that infants are even more determined to accomplish a goal. However, they are still developmentally dependent and the disconnect between their motor abilities, their communication skills, and their wants can create great frustration for the infants. Although there are early signs of foundational language, such as stringing together sounds like "da-da," it is far from what is needed to express emotion, so 9- and 12-month-olds revert to crying for communication. For example, a common condition that infants struggle to communicate is teething pain, so outward drooling, fussiness, and frustration may be the only signs of primary tooth eruption.

Exploration, Exuberance, and Early Childhood (15–24 Months Old)

This stage may very well be the most developmentally explosive of all the stages. Physically, growth is somewhat stable, but there is great refinement in the gross and fine motor skills. Toddlers build their independence and begin walking and running between activities, exploring previously uninteresting corners and cabinets of the house, and explaining their findings with an expanding vocabulary. Their play moves from playing alone to playing in parallel with other toddlers, but stranger apprehension may have them hiding behind their mothers' legs in unfamiliar situations.

Funny, Fickle, and Friendly (3 Years Old)

Having gained great motor control, the 3-year-old has developed the coordination to ride a tricycle, dress and undress herself, draw with some precision, and prepare a bowl of cereal. She understands two-step commands and has an extensive vocabulary that is 75% understandable. She has begun to learn to take turns, making interactive play easier to facilitate. At this stage, children crave attention and will use their new-found vocabulary and growing intelligence to say funny things to make adults laugh. They make friends easily, yet they can be fickle about foods, sleep, and being offered help with daily tasks. Meltdowns are not uncommon.

Gregarious, Goofy, and Getting Ready (4 Years Old)

Four-year-olds are "big kids" with big imaginations. Physically, their growth continues at a modest pace, but their coordination is improving. They typically attend preschool and are beginning to recognize letters and sounds, print their names with a mature pencil grasp, draw pictures, and play collaboratively with friends. They may ride a bike with training wheels and are the gregarious, "who, what, when, and why" kids with insatiable curiosity. Their magical thinking brings imaginary friends to life and goofy details to a story. Their daily play and experiential learning are getting them ready for formal learning in kindergarten.

Honing, Habits, and Heading Off to School (5–6 Years Old)

This stage marks a dramatic shift in development from primarily outward development to more cognitive development. The visual difference between the first day and the last day of kindergarten may be only a few inches or pounds, but the cognitive changes are tremendous. School-aged children must undertake cognitive and psychosocial tasks to have educational and social achievement and must shift from "taking it all in" to differentiating between important and unimportant information. The kindergartener must hone their self-regulation, exhibit impulse control, follow the rules, and make friends. There is also a shift from isolated developmental tasks to activities that require integration of multiple skills, such as sitting still, following directions, managing time, and sequencing the execution of a task, which requires persistence and sustained attention. The most successful school-aged learners are those who have healthy, productive habits modeled and reinforced, both at home and in the school environment.

When they are not in school, they love to climb trees, hop and skip, ride a bike, and practice printing with improved precision. They play cooperatively with others and may even join their first sports team. They show off their counting skills and letter decoding, as they learn simple arithmetic and reading.

Independent, Inventive, and Inquisitive (7–10 Years Old)

Well established in school routines, 7- to 10-year-olds have now made the transition to school life, gained small doses of independence, and improved simple executive functions. They have also transitioned from a learning-to-read stage to a reading-to-learn mindset. School performance has become the developmental gauge. This is also the time that learning disabilities and attention-deficit hyperactivity disorder (ADHD) may become apparent, so inquiring about school performance, inability to keep up with grade-level expectations or teacher concerns can uncover these issues. Same-gender friendships and activities that require increased coordination and physical skill dominate the inventive playground games at recess. The elementary school child has slow and steady growth and by age 10 may exhibit some early pubertal changes, such as body odor, increased oil production on the facial skin, axillary hair, and acne (blackheads and pimples). This increases modesty and may change the dynamic of the WCC (e.g., draping appropriately during exam, asking siblings to step out of room, and giving choice to talk with provider alone).

Junior High Journey, Judgment, and Juggling Change (11–12 Years Old)

The physical and social-emotional changes associated with tweens are some of the most dramatic since the toddler years. Although girls may begin some early pubertal changes between 9 and 10 years old, the majority of the hormonal and physical changes occur in the tween years, whereas boys tend to lag behind by a year or two. Puberty, like other developmental phases, follows a fairly predictable pattern for both males and females. Although predictable for practitioners, the changes associated with menstruation or nocturnal emissions are anything but comfortable or predictable for the tween. Equally difficult for some tweens is understanding their gender identity and sexual orientation. For some, the physical changes associated with puberty do not align with their identity or their attractions do not align with societal norms.

Rapid growth and physical changes create an increased nutritional demand, a shift in sleep cycles, increasing myelination of the brain's frontal lobe and emotional lability. The middle school or junior high patient can appear distracted, introverted, or may be difficult to engage in conversation. Practitioners who see tweens and teens often use the mnemonic HEEADSS (home, education, eating, activities, drugs, sexuality, suicidality) as a framework for how to approach the interview with these patients. Starting with the topics that are more comfortable (home life and school) and moving toward those that might cause more uneasiness for teens (sexuality, substance abuse and mood) allows the provider to ease the patient into the conversation, and it helps to build rapport for tackling some of the tougher questions. As demonstrated in the sample note on page 20, the concepts from NEST & FLY parallel the HEEADSS mnemonic so either one can be useful when working with adolescents. If you are able to put the tween at ease in the office, you may find a very egocentric, "the world revolves around me" perspective, short-sighted thinking, and an invincibility that could put him into risky situations. It is possible that just a look, questioning her thinking, or even a compliment can leave her feeling judged by adults who "don't understand."

Knee-Jerk Reactions, Kindred Connections, and Keeping Up (13–14 Years Old)

The early teen years can be especially difficult from a social-emotional perspective, as the brain's center for emotional regulation is still in its infancy, yet physically both boys and girls are usually somewhere along the pubertal spectrum and in various stages of physical change. The immature emotional epicenter leads to knee-jerk reactions and poorly planned actions that can become problematic at both home and school. There is also a continuum when it comes to self-awareness about sexual orientation. Many early adolescents waver between confident and confused when trying to understand their sexual attractions. Adjusting to increased responsibility and independence, burgeoning love interests, and climbing school demands can be daunting for early teens. Add on trying to create their own identity, find a peer group that they can relate to, and grapple with their burgeoning abstract thinking, it is no wonder that some teens begin to struggle with anxiety and depression during this time. Early to middle adolescents experiment with appearance via hairstyles, clothing, jewelry, makeup, and piercings, all in an effort to overcome self-consciousness, "fit in," and find their clan.

Love, Licenses, and Life After High School (15–18 Years Old)

At 15 to 18 years old, teens are now making their way through the halls of high school trying to navigate the unstable landscape of social status, romantic relationships, and increasing independence. Toward the later end of this stage, teens are preparing for life after high school, whether that be working, going to college, or attending a trade school. Although much of the physical change of puberty is complete by 15, patients' outward appearances and brain development continue to morph until their mid-20s, which means they are developing the ability to make judgments using sound reasoning but may resort to more emotional decision-making when put in pressured situations. These emotional decisions continue to lead to risk-taking behaviors, especially as related to sexual exploration, illegal substances, and driving. However, these middle adolescents do not respond well to a preaching approach, but rather want to be engaged in open discussions and eventually be allowed to make their own decisions.

The thorough head-to-toe assessment associated with the WCC pays particular attention to age-appropriate physical exam findings that may herald a problem with growth or development. As these vary by age, specific standout components will be included in the charts at the heart of this pocket guide.

Special care has been taken to include the components of a thorough pre-participation sports evaluation, the physical exam maneuvers, and what abnormal findings could indicate.

The sports physical or pre-participation exam may be one of the few entry points into the healthcare system for school-aged and adolescent patients, and it presents unique challenges from a history and physical exam perspective. The goals of the visit are fourfold and include the following:

1. Assessing the athlete's fitness level for a specific sport or activity

2. Identifying medical or orthopedic problems that may put the athlete at risk for illness, injury, or impaired performance

3. Meeting legal and insurance requirements of the school district or other agency

4. Supplying education on sports safety to maintain the health and safety of the athlete, age-appropriate exercise, injury prevention, and other health-related issues

The NEST & FLY mnemonic can still be applied to this specific type of pediatric visit, but some of the components of the NEST & FLY mnemonic do change. Although not exemplar, sometimes these visits are done outside of a medical home so there are not data points to track longitudinally. For this reason, instead of tracking, the NEST focus turns to *Timing*. Ideally, the PPE should be performed with enough time for referrals, preseason conditioning, and injury rehabilitation should those be necessary. As for the FLY portion of the mnemonic, family is still an important component of the history; however, a focused family, past medical, and sports-specific history are the *Facts* that play the biggest role in determining restrictions and the need for further evaluation. *Level of contact* and the static versus dynamic nature of the activities the athlete intends to participate in can also influence a clearance decision. *Your tools* continue to include a thorough physical exam that is modified to detect common cardiovascular and orthopedic issues that may not be uncovered with the history alone, whereas anticipatory guidance is important in helping the athlete maintain good health and prevent injuries.

Screening and diagnostic tests are part of your toolbox, which allow you to investigate for congenital diseases, micronutrient deficiency, heavy-metal poisoning, developmental delays, autism, high-risk behaviors, infectious diseases, and depression. In accordance with the AAP Committee on Practice and Ambulatory Medicine policy recommendations, they will be indicated in the charts.[14]

One of the most useful resources available to support your observations and developmental surveillance are screening questionnaires. These questionnaires screen for delays in development, emotional and behavioral symptoms, family stress, autism spectrum disorder, substance use, and depression. Table 1 lists some commonly used tools and their screening functions.

As every practice is different and visits need to be tailored to the needs of the family and child, not all the suggested screenings may be appropriate.

Table 1: Commonly Used Screening Questionnaires*

Questionnaire Name and Abbreviation		Validated Ages	What It Screens For
Ages and Stages Questionnaires®	ASQ®	2 months to 5 years	Delays in gross and fine motor skills, communication, problem-solving, adaptive behaviors
Modified Checklist for Autism in Toddlers™	M-CHAT™	16–30 months	Autism spectrum disorder
Pediatric Evaluation of Developmental Status	PEDS	Birth to 8 years	Problems with language, motor skills, early academic skills, behavior, and social-emotional, mental health
Pediatric Symptom Checklist	PSC	4–16 years	Emotional and behavioral problems
Strengths and Difficulties Questionnaires	SDQ	3–16 years	Emotional symptoms, conduct problems, hyperactivity, inattention, peer problems, and prosocial behaviors
Survey of Well-Being of Young Children	SWYC	2 months to 5 years	Delays in cognitive, motor, and language development
Baby Pediatric Symptom Checklist	BPSC	2–18 months	Irritability, inflexibility, and difficulty with routines
Preschool Pediatric Symptom Checklist	PPSC	18–66 months	Behavior
Parent's Observations of Social Interactions	POSI	18–35 months	Autism spectrum disorder
Brief Screener for Tobacco, Alcohol, and Other Drugs	BSTAD	12–17 years	Tobacco, alcohol, and marijuana use
Car, Relax, Alone, Forget, Friends, Trouble	CRAFFT	Adolescents	Substance use
Edinburgh Postnatal Depression Scale	EPDS	Peripartum women	Postpartum depression
Patient Health Questionnaire+	PHQ	>11 years	Depression
Abuse Assessment Screen	AAS	Adolescent or adult	Interpersonal violence
Health Leads Screening		All ages	Food insecurity, housing instability, utility needs, transportation troubles, violence exposures, demographics
Pediatric ACEs and Related Life-Events Screener	PEARLS	0–19 years^	Abuse, neglect, and household challenges (growing up in a household with incarceration, mental illness, substance dependence, absence due to separation or divorce, or IPV)

*This list is not comprehensive and should not be seen as endorsement of one particular tool over others not listed.
+Available in 9-question adolescent or a 2- or 9-question adult versions.
^Caregiver-completed tool for ages 0–19 years and adolescent self-report tool for 12–19 years.

Completing the WCC should include discussing those issues that a parent or patient can anticipate by the next visit, those issues that can affect growth or development, or those issues of question or concern. As a large part of the anticipatory guidance in pediatrics focuses on safety and health, it is no surprise that immunizations fall into this category as well.

Immunizations

The current vaccination schedule used in the United States includes infant vaccinations for diphtheria, tetanus, and acellular pertussis (DTaP), *Haemophilus influenzae* type b (Hib), hepatitis B (HepB), influenza (IIV), pneumococcal (PCV13), inactivated poliovirus (IPV), and rotavirus (RV).[15]

Many of the infant vaccinations require booster vaccinations in childhood. After the first birthday, there is also the introduction of vaccinations for hepatitis A (HepA), measles, mumps and rubella (MMR), and varicella (VAR).[15]

Beginning at 11 years old, adolescents should be offered those vaccinations exclusive to preadolescent and adolescent patients, including human papillomavirus (HPV), meningococcal serogroup A, C, W, Y (MenACWY), meningococcal serogroup B (MenB), and tetanus, diphtheria, and acellular pertussis (Tdap).[15]

Table 2 outlines the most commonly used immunization schedule at the recommended ages; however, for the most current updates and footnotes, referring to the Advisory Committee on Immunization Practices (ACIP) or Centers for Disease Control and Prevention (CDC) websites is wise.

Table 3 can be used to determine the dose of pain reliever the child can be given should the immunizations cause myalgias or a low-grade temperature.

Anticipatory Guidance

When given the opportunity to observe birds in the wild, it is not surprising that NESTS serve as the hub from which they chirp, sing, and educate their young. Similarly, you can think about your anticipatory guidance as educating patients and families about NESTS (**N**utrition, **E**xercise [or Elimination], **S**leep, **T**rajectories for growth and development, and **S**afety).

Table 2: Vaccine Schedule by Most Commonly Administered WCC Ages

Vaccine	Birth	2 months	4 months	6 months	12–15 months	15–18 months	24 months	4–5 years	11–12 years	15–16 years
DTaP		#1	#2	#3		#4		#5		
HepA					#1	#2^				
HepB	#1	#2		#3						
Hib		#1	#2	#3*	#4					
HPV									#1 and #2	
IPV		#1	#2	#3				#4		
MenACWY									#1	#2
MenB										#1, #2, #3*
MMR					#1			#2		
PCV13		#1	#2	#3	#4					
RV		#1	#2	#3*						
Tdap									#1	
VAR					#1			#2		
IIV				Once annually after 2-dose season (starting after 6 months of age)						

*Dose may be necessary depending on the vaccine used.
^If >6 months since the first dose.
Modified from CDC Immunization Schedules.[15]

Table 3: Dosing Recommendations for Acetaminophen and Ibuprofen

Acetaminophen Infant and children liquid suspension (160 mg/5 mL) Chewable tablets (80 mg, 160 mg^) Adult regular strength capsules or tablets (325 mg) Adult extra strength capsules or tablets (500 mg)		Ibuprofen Infant drops (50 mg/1.25 mL) Children's liquid suspension (100 mg/5 mL) Chewable tablets (100 mg) Junior-strength tablets (100 mg) Adult-strength tablets (200 mg)
Weight (lbs)	**Amount to give (mg)**	**Amount to give (mg)**
6–11	40 mg (1.25 mL liquid)	Not approved for under 6 months of age or 11 pounds
12–17	80 mg (2.5 mL liquid)	50 mg (1.25 mL infant drops OR 2.5 mL liquid)
18–23	120 mg (3.75 mL liquid OR 1 ½ chewable tablets)	75 mg (1.875 mL infant drops OR 4 mL liquid)
24–35	160 mg (5 mL liquid OR 1 chewable tablet)	100 mg (2.5 mL infant drops OR 5 mL liquid OR 1 chewable tablet)
36–47	240 mg (7.5 mL liquid OR 1 ½ chewable tablets)	150 mg (3.75 mL infant drops OR 7.5 mL liquid OR 1.5 chewable tablets)
48–59	325 mg (10 mL liquid OR 2 chewable tablets OR 1 regular strength)	200 mg (5 mL infant drops OR 10 mL liquid OR 2 chewable tablets OR 2 junior-strength tablets OR 1 adult-strength tablets)
60–71	400 mg (12.5 mL liquid OR 2 ½ chewable tablets OR 1 regular strength)	250 mg (12.5 mL liquid OR 2.5 chewable tablets OR 2.5 junior-strength tablets OR 1 adult-strength tablet)
72–95	480 mg (15 mL liquid OR 3 chewable tablets OR 1 ½ regular strength OR 1 extra strength)	300 mg (15 mL liquid OR 3 chewable tablets OR 3 junior-strength tablets OR 1 ½ adult-strength tablets)
≥96	650 mg (20 mL liquid OR 4 chewable tablets OR 2 regular strength OR 1 extra strength)	400 mg (20 mL liquid OR 4 chewable tablets OR 4 junior-strength tablets OR 2 adult-strength tablets)

*Dosing for preterm and term neonates (0–29 days) is calculated using different dosing assumptions.
^Tylenol® only manufactures 160 mg tablets, but other manufacturers may still be offering 80 mg tablets, so it is important to verify the dose the parent is using prior to providing dosing directions.

DOCUMENTING THE WELL VISIT

With the growth of electronic health records (EHRs), documentation of the well visit has become more dependent on the system and the clinic guidelines set for providers; however, using the concepts of NEST & FLY in your documentation can help streamline and standardize your documentation across ages and stages.

Boxes 2 to 4 show examples of an infant, school-aged, and adolescent note in a modified SOAP format. However, it is important to recognize that these components may vary depending on the templating of your particular EHR.

BOX 2: SAMPLE DOCUMENTATION FOR INFANT WELL-CHILD EXAM

Infant A is a 2-month-old female

NUTRITION
- Breastfeeding q2–3 hours during the day for 10–15 minutes/side and q3–5 hours at night with complete resolution of engorgement after feeding. Mother continues on prenatal vitamins and well-balanced diet that includes three glasses of milk daily, and infant is receiving 400 IU of vitamin D QD via dropper. No supplemental feedings provided

ELIMINATION
- Eliminates q2–3 days with yellow seedy stools and urinates with almost every feed

SLEEP
- Sleeps for 2–2.5 hour stretches 2–3× during day and has longest stretch at night (5 hours). Typically falls asleep at the breast. Caregivers put her back to sleep in crib for naps with swaddling and pacifier

TRACKING
- Growth at 25th percentile for length, weight, and HC

FAMILY
- Parents returning to work full-time this month, so Infant A will be attending day care 3×/week and 2×/week with paternal grandmother
- Financially stable and does not qualify for supplemental assistance programs
- No secondhand smoke in the home

LEARNING/DEVELOPMENT
- No concerns about development from parents
- Beginning to coo and smile; recognizes faces; brings hands to midline; bicycling legs; no rolling yet, but lifts head when prone

YOUR TOOLS
- Post-partum depression screen for mother—4 (negative)

PHYSICAL EXAM
WD/WN female with NC/AT head. AFOSF with no bulging. EOMI with movement past midline in horizontal, nares patent, O/P clear with no evidence of thrust, cleft, or ankyloglossia. Neck is supple with mild head lag on pulling to sit. Lungs CTA bilaterally and CV with no murmurs. 2+FP×2, <2 sec. cap refill. Abdomen is S/NT/ND. No hernias. Negative O/B, equal leg lengths with symmetric leg skin folds, +Moro, suck, palmar grasp, Galant and Babinski reflexes. Rooting reflex resolved. Hearing is grossly intact. Normal female genitalia

IMMUNIZATIONS
HepB#2 Rota #1 PCV#1
Hib #1 DTaP#1 IPV#1

ASSESSMENT
Healthy 2-month-old female with stable and concordant growth at the 25th percentile and age-appropriate development

PLAN & ANTICIPATORY GUIDANCE
- Recommended next well visit at 4 months of age
- Encouraged continued exclusive breastfeeding and discussed challenges to anticipate with pumping and returning to work
- Reviewed expected changes in stooling patterns for BF infants
- Sleep patterns to become routine and sleep times to lengthen
- Expect growth trajectory to continue along the 10th–50th percentile
- Discussed resources for talking with caregivers about what to do when stressed with an infant and to "never shake a baby"
- Encouraged date night once a month, if possible
- Anticipated milestones reviewed, tummy time encouraged, importance of early literacy introduction reviewed

BOX 3: SAMPLE DOCUMENTATION FOR SCHOOL-AGED WELL-CHILD EXAM

Child A is an 8-year-old male accompanied by his caregiver

NUTRITION
- Eats 3 meals a day—2 at school through the national breakfast and lunch program and 1 at home. Occasional food scarcity, but maternal grandmother (MGM) uses the food pantry at the church when needed. Canned and frozen fruits and veggies. Favorite is apples. Minimal meats (1–2×/week)—chicken. + pasta. No vitamins. Whole wheat bread for sandwiches, but not pasta. Eats fast food 3–4 times a week. Milk with school lunch. Brushing teeth 2×/day; saw dentist 2 months ago

EXERCISE
- PE class 2–3×/week for 75 minutes. Recess 2×/day for 30 minutes. No organized sports. 3+ hours of video/TV on weekdays

SLEEP
- Sleeps with younger brother. Top bunk. Bedtime is 8:30 p.m. Wakes at 6:30 a.m. No snoring per caregiver

TRACKING
- Growth at 50th percentile for height, weight, and BMI

FAMILY
- Lives with MGM, mother, uncle, and younger brother in apartment. Mother works nights at hospital as phlebotomist
- Financially stretched at times. Qualifies for WIC for younger brother, SNAP benefits, and state CHIP
- No secondhand smoke in the home, but + in apartment building

LEARNING/DEVELOPMENT
- He attends Lincoln Elementary School and is in the 3rd grade
- At grade level in reading, but behind in math
- No IEP or 504b

YOUR TOOLS
- Snellen exam: 20/30 (R) and 20/25 (L), hearing intact

PHYSICAL EXAM
Well appearing male, cooperative, polite. NC/AT; PERRL, EOMI, (–) Hirschberg test, conjunctiva clear; O/P clear with 1+ tonsils. Fillings noted on back pre-molars. Newly erupting lateral incisors and fully erupted central incisors. Nares clear. TMs partially obstructed by soft cerumen but pearly gray. Neck with no thyromegaly. Lungs CTA bilaterally and CV with no murmurs. 2+FP bilaterally, <2 seconds cap refill. Abdomen is S/NT/ND, but ticklish. Normal gait and balance with 5/5 strength in UE and LE; Tanner I circumcised male with bilateral testicles

IMMUNIZATIONS
Influenza (annual); up to date on childhood immunizations

ASSESSMENT
Healthy 8-year-old male with stable growth at the 50th percentile, despite intermittent financial and food insecurity. Developmentally, meeting grade-level expectations in literacy but below grade-level in math

PLAN & ANTICIPATORY GUIDANCE
- Recommended next well visit in 1 year
- Discussed school performance. Making progress in math, so will watch but if continues to fall behind, consider evaluation for LD
- Encouraged continued use of food assistance programs and cookbook on kid-friendly foods on a budget given to the family Start daily MV given low vitamin D, calcium, and iron intake
- Discussed canned fruit in water (not syrup) and frozen veggies
- Discussed recommendations for <2 hours of screen time/day and 1 hour of activity a day. Handout on rec center sports given to family
- Continue to work for 10–11 hours of sleep/night
- Reviewed growth and expected to continue along 50th percentile

BOX 4: SAMPLE DOCUMENTATION FOR ADOLESCENT WELL-CHILD EXAM (USING BOTH NEST AND HEEADSS MNEMONICS)

Teen A is a 14-year-old female here with mom, who is in waiting area

NUTRITION
- Skips breakfast (1–2×/week) when late for school. Fruit smoothies in AM. School lunch but doesn't eat a lot because "we don't have much time." Fruit or granola bar before golf practice. Meat (only chicken) 1–3×/week, but eggs almost daily. +wheat bread, Raisin Bran sometimes. 1 glass of milk/day + MV with calcium. Routine dentist/orthodontist

EXERCISE
- On golf team, so playing 5–6×/week. Has PE class (dance) as well

SLEEP
- Sleeps "pretty good." Goes to bed at 9:00 p.m.; wakes at 5:30 a.m.
- No trouble falling asleep or staying asleep. Phone in room, but ringer off at night

TRACKING
- Height stable at 5'4" × 2 years. Weight up 4 pounds. BMI at 35th percentile

FAMILY (HOME AND EMPLOYMENT)
- Lives with both parents and 1 younger brother. No secondhand smoke
- Can talk to dad more than mom but pretty open relationship with both
- Has some chores/responsibilities but also has privacy/own room
- Family financially stable; teen not working

LEARNING (EDUCATION AND ACTIVITIES)
- Freshman at Jefferson HS. Honors courses. Group of three friends
- Involved in school musical and band; <3 hours of leisure screen time

YOUR TOOLS (DRUGS, SEXUALITY, SUICIDE)
- PHQ-9-4; CRAFFT-0 → Denies drug, alcohol or marijuana use
- Boyfriend × 1 year (–) sexually active and not planning. (+) OCPs—acne
- Sometimes feels down about school/self-expectations but denies depression/anxiety or suicidality

PHYSICAL EXAM
WD/WN female with bubbly affect. NC/AT; PERRL, EOMI, conjunctiva clear; O/P clear. +braces. Nares clear. TMs pearly gray. Neck supple, no thyromegaly. Lungs CTA bilaterally and CV exam with no murmurs on sitting, standing or with Valsalva. <2 sec. cap refill. Abdomen is S/NT/ND, no organomegaly, umbilical piercing. Normal gait and balance with symmetric duck walk, no ankle or knee instability; Tanner IV female breasts, and pubic hair

IMMUNIZATIONS
Influenza (annual); up to date on Tdap, meningococcal, and HPV vaccines

ASSESSMENT
Healthy 14-year-old female with stable height and BMI Developmentally appropriate at Tanner IV. Low-risk adolescent with negative depression and substance abuse screens

PLAN & ANTICIPATORY GUIDANCE
- Recommended next well visit in 1 year
- Encouraged packing lunch night before and some recipes for quick grab-and-go breakfast options when in a hurry
- Provided daily exercise and plan for exercise when golf season is over
- Discussed sleep hygiene principles
- Advised patient she has reached adult height, but minor changes in pubertal development will continue over the next year
- Gave student information on LARC for future planning
- Reviewed techniques to handle peer pressure around high-risk behaviors and encouraged patient to talk with trusted adult if feeling sad, depressed, overwhelmed, or anxious
- Seatbelts, sunscreen, and bike safety also reviewed

Newborn (3–5 Days Old)

NUTRITION

NATURAL FOODS:	Exclusive breastfeeding recommended; primarily colostrum for first 3–5 days; iron-fortified formula is alternative • Breastfeeding: 8–10×/day at 10–20 minutes per side; may fall asleep at the breast • Bottle feeding: 6–8 feeds/day; average is 30–32 oz/day
VITAMINS:	Vitamin D (400 IU) daily if breastfeeding[16] and prenatal vitamins for breastfeeding mother
IRON SOURCES:	Iron stores typically sufficient in term infant Iron found in breast milk (lactoferrin) is highly bioavailable, so no supplement needed if exclusively breastfeeding[10]
GRAINS:	Ask about maternal diet and encourage high-fiber diet to help with maternal constipation
ADDED SUGAR/SALT:	Ask about maternal diet Encourage healthy diet for mother with minimal salt to help with reducing fluid retention
TEETH:	Assess for presence of natal teeth. If present, refer to pediatric dentist for removal (to prevent possible choking hazard) Ask about mother's last dental visit; encourage routine oral health care to prevent early childhood caries later in child's life
DAIRY:	Breast milk or formula

ELIMINATION

URINATION:	6–8 wet diapers/day
STOOLING:	Breastfed: 1–4 transitional to yellow, seedy stools[17] · Formula fed: Transitional stools; 1–2/day

SLEEP

POSITION:	Put on back for sleeping[18]
QUANTITY:	4–5 hour stretch may be the longest at night; 3–4 naps of 2–4 hours; total: 16–18 hours
ROUTINE:	Baby should be laid in bassinet or crib before falling asleep when possible, but often falls asleep at breast or with bottle Expect nighttime awakenings for both breastfed and bottle-fed babies No pacifier use until breastfeeding well established
SLEEP SITE & SAFETY:	AAP recommends co-sleeper, bassinet, or crib with room sharing; no bed sharing[18] Snug mattress and narrow crib slats in crib; no bottles, plush toys, blankets, pillows, bumpers in sleeping area

TRACKING

GROWTH:	Should have <10% birth weight loss with some upward trend in weight once mother's milk supply comes in[10,19] Difficult to note significant changes in length and HC from birth at this visit
INTERVAL HISTORY:	Review the prenatal and birth history, nursery course, and routine interventions done in the newborn nursery Ask about birth and hospital experience

FAMILY

Family, Including Siblings & Outside Supports:	Introduction to the family (who lives in the house, including siblings, pets, and extended family members) Type of housing and transportation Ask about specific challenges for the family
	Query about support networks (e.g., family, friends)
Adjustment to Age or Stage:	Screen for baby blues New responsibilities New baby in the home
Money:	Establish employment, housing, and financial barriers Offer community resources to help with insurance or government health plan enrollment for infant, if needed Ensure that parent/guardian has a primary care provider of their own, should an issue need to be addressed in the future
Safety:	Review prenatal history with specific focus on interpersonal violence during pregnancy Ask about secondhand smoke, vaping, THC exposure

LEARNING

Physical Development

Gross Motor:	Limited vision with poor eye control Suck, swallow, breathe without difficulties Moves all extremities Infantile reflexes	**Fine Motor:**	None to note

Communication/Language Development

Verbal:	None to note	**Nonverbal:**	Undifferentiated cry Cry that is weak vs. strong

Cognitive/Intellectual Development

Intelligence:	None to note	**Problem-Solving:**	Note to note

Social–Emotional Development

Connection:	Sustains periods of wakefulness for feedings Fixes briefly on faces or objects Follows face to midline	**Self-Regulation:**	Possibly thumb-sucking

YOUR TOOLS	
YOUR INTERVIEW:	*Tell me about how breastfeeding is going. What signs tell you that your baby is hungry? How do you know that your baby is satisfied?* Ask about sore nipples, sensations of engorgement, sensations of letdown, changes in milk color/quantity. *Tell me about your sleep schedule the last couple of days (e.g., what is the longest stretch of sleep you've been able to get?).* *How many wet diapers and stool diapers is the baby having per day?*
YOUR OBSERVATIONS:	When awake, the infant should be alert but may be sleeping upon exam with an irregular breathing pattern. Caregiver engagement, excitement, and anxiety may be noticeable, or you may have to ask how mom is sleeping, eating, feeling, and behaving, as this may not be information given without prompting.

PHYSICAL EXAM:		COMPLETE PHYSICAL EXAM WITH A SPECIFIC FOCUS ON	NORMAL FINDINGS SOMETIMES SEEN AT THIS AGE
	HEAD:	Palpate fontanelles and skull Evaluate for caput or cephalohematoma	Anterior and posterior fontanelles are open, soft, flat; sutures could be split or slightly overriding; molding
	EYES:	Note red reflexes and assess for fixation Assess for conjunctival injection or discharge	Uncoordinated eye movements Blinks in response to bright light or touching eye[20]
	EARS:	Note position, malformation	Lop ear deformity; preauricular ear tag or skin pits[21]
	NECK:	Assess for clavicular crepitus and torticollis	No head control
	MOUTH:	Inspect uvula, palate, tongue, frenulum, and gums	Epstein pearls[22]
	CHEST:	Auscultate for murmurs, adventitious lung sounds	Enlargement of breast tissue; milky breast discharge
	ABDOMEN:	Palpate for masses, defects, HSM Palpate femoral pulses bilaterally	Umbilical cord still on; diastasis rectus
	MSK/NEURO:	Perform Ortolani and Barlow maneuvers Assess tone, leg length, and skin fold symmetry	
	REFLEXES:	Rooting, suck, Moro, and Babinski reflexes	(+) Babinski
	GENITALIA:	Inspect for clitoral enlargement (♀), microphallus (♂), urethral and testicular position (♂) Note circumcision status and patency of anus	Pseudomenses and vaginal tag (♀)[23] Epidermal cyst at the tip of foreskin (♂)[23] Hydrocele, as determined by transillumination
	SKIN:	Jaundice, lesions, rashes, bruising, birthmarks	Peeling skin; lanugo; salmon patch; congenital dermal melanocytosis (previously called Mongolian spots); acrocyanosis; pustules or collarette of scale from transient neonatal pustular melanosis; erythema toxicum; harlequin color change[24]

<table>
<tr><td colspan="3" align="center">YOUR TOOLS</td></tr>
<tr><td align="right">Screenings:</td><td colspan="2">Hearing screen (if not done prior to hospital discharge or if the child failed newborn hearing screen)</td></tr>
<tr><td align="right">Immunizations:</td><td colspan="2">HepB (if not given in the hospital)</td></tr>
<tr><td rowspan="5">Anticipatory Guidance:</td><td colspan="2" align="center">Baby Joys, Baby Blues, and Breastfeeding (the First Month of Life)
Anticipatory guidance at this age centers on the 3 Bs—breast/bottle feeding, breathing, and beds</td></tr>
<tr><td align="right">Nutrition:</td><td>Continue to offer breast milk (or formula) as the sole nutrition source; feed 8–12 times in a 24-hour period based on hunger cues
Educate mothers on the changes that occur at the breast with continued breastfeeding, such as less engorgement, milk being made on demand with suckling, milk composition changes throughout a feeding, less letdown sensation
Prescribe vitamin D 400 IU daily, if breastfeeding babies are not currently using
If offering formula, make a fresh bottle with every feeding (1 scoop formula for every 2 oz of water). Encourage paced-bottle feeding, so infant controls flow and intake</td></tr>
<tr><td align="right">Elimination:</td><td>Breastfeeding stools will change to soft, yellow, and seedy with exclusive breastfeeding; will likely continue with several per day until 2-week visit
Formula-fed infants have brown to tan stools; will likely continue with 1–2/day until 2-week visit</td></tr>
<tr><td align="right">Sleep:</td><td>Sleep will continue to be primary activity but should be able to arouse for feeds
SIDS reduction practices should be reviewed (i.e., swaddling, put back to sleep in a crib or co-sleeper, no bed sharing, no secondhand smoke exposure)</td></tr>
<tr><td align="right">Trajectory:</td><td>Infant breathing patterns begin to become more regular
Growth expectations → Gain about 1 oz/day
Upcoming milestones → Increasing periods of wakefulness; more regular sleep patterns</td></tr>
<tr><td></td><td align="right">Safety:</td><td>Turn hot water heater to <120° and always test water temperature prior to placing infant in bath
Car seat should be a 5-point harness, backward-facing infant carrier in the back seat
No use of infant swings until baby is able to hold neck stable
Review postpartum depression symptoms
Prepare for increasing episodes of infant crying and offer some techniques to handle (e.g., swaddling, pacifier use, infant massage, skin-to-skin care, car rides, etc.)</td></tr>
</table>

NUTRITION

Natural Foods:	Exclusive breastfeeding recommended; milk supply being established in first 2–3 weeks of life; breast milk composition varies throughout a feeding with increasing fat after initial thirst/hunger satisfied[10] Iron-fortified formula is alternative • Breastfeeding: 8–10×/day at 10–20 minutes per side • Bottle feeding: 6–8 feeds/day; 30–32 oz/day
Vitamins:	Vitamin D (400 IU) daily if breastfeeding and prenatal vitamins for breastfeeding mother
Iron Sources:	Iron found in breast milk (lactoferrin) is highly bioavailable, so no supplement needed Use iron-fortified formula if supplementing or not breastfeeding
Grains:	Breastfeeding mother should be eating a high-fiber diet to help with possible maternal constipation
Added Sugar/Salt:	Ask about maternal diet Encourage healthy diet with minimal salt to help with reducing fluid retention
Teeth:	Ask about last routine dental visit for mother; encourage routine oral health care as a means of preventing early childhood caries later in child's life
Dairy:	Breast milk or formula

ELIMINATION

Urination:	4–6 wet diapers/day
Stooling:	Breastfed: 4 yellow, loose, seedy stool diapers — Formula fed: Tan to brown; 3–4/day

SLEEP

Position:	Put on back for sleeping
Quantity:	4-hour stretch at night may be the longest; numerous naps throughout day; total: 16–18 hours
Routine:	More frequent nighttime awakenings for breastfed babies If swaddling, ensure knees can bend up and out; monitor for overheating Pacifier use OK for sleep after breastfeeding well established (usually around 3–4 weeks); should not use throughout day
Sleep Site & Safety:	AAP recommends co-sleeper or crib with room sharing; no bed sharing Snug mattress and narrow crib slats in crib No bottles, plush toys, blankets, pillows, bumpers in sleeping area

TRACKING

Growth:	Infant should have regained birth weight by 2 weeks and begin gaining ~1 oz/day until 2 months May see a slight change (larger or smaller) in HC, as molding, sutures, and any birth traumas begin to resolve

NEWBORNS

2 Weeks to 1 Month

FAMILY

FAMILY, INCLUDING SIBLINGS & OUTSIDE SUPPORTS:	Division of responsibility (who bathes, who changes infant at night, who warms bottles, etc.) Inquire about sibling response to the new baby Ask about support networks (e.g., family, friends, etc.) Review childcare plans, if parent returning to work and respite care supports, if staying at home
ADJUSTMENT TO AGE OR STAGE:	Maternal sleep patterns Feeding routines Having a new baby in the home
MONEY:	Discuss plans to return to work, including length of family leave Refer to WIC program for nutritional supplement, if needed and qualify
SAFETY:	Ask about secondhand smoke, vaping, THC exposure Discuss safety plan for crying infant Screen for maternal depression

LEARNING

PHYSICAL DEVELOPMENT

GROSS MOTOR:	Limited vision with poor eye control Suck, swallow, breathe without difficulties Moves all extremities Infantile reflexes	**FINE MOTOR:**	None to note

COMMUNICATION/LANGUAGE DEVELOPMENT

VERBAL:	None to note	**NONVERBAL:**	Undifferentiated cry Communicates needs via behaviors

COGNITIVE/INTELLECTUAL DEVELOPMENT

INTELLIGENCE:	None to note	**PROBLEM-SOLVING:**	Note to note

SOCIAL–EMOTIONAL DEVELOPMENT

CONNECTION:	Has some regard for surroundings Fixes briefly on faces or objects Follows faces to midline	**SELF-REGULATION:**	Thumb-sucking for soothing

YOUR TOOLS		
YOUR INTERVIEW:	*Tell me about how breastfeeding is going. How do you know when baby is satisfied? What does your feeding routine or schedule look like during a 24-hour period?* *Tell me about your sleep schedule.*	
YOUR OBSERVATIONS:	There should be signs of a bond forming between the baby and her caregiver(s), with the caregiver responding to the infant's needs promptly and with gentleness and flexibility. Because it may not always be outwardly obvious, asking about signs of maternal postpartum depression can provide important clues to family functioning, responsiveness, and attachment.	
PHYSICAL EXAM:	**COMPLETE PHYSICAL EXAM WITH A SPECIFIC FOCUS ON**	**NORMAL FINDINGS YOU MIGHT SEE AT THIS AGE**
	HEAD: Palpate fontanelles	Anterior fontanelle and posterior fontanelle both palpable, soft, and flat
	EYES: Note red reflexes Assess for fixation and alignment	Poor tracking, but if it occurs, infant may not track across midline Intermittent strabismus No pupillary response
	NECK: Assess for masses, shortening of clavicle, and/or torticollis	Head lag
	MOUTH: Inspect buccal mucosa, uvula, palate, tongue, frenulum, and gums	Epstein pearls; Bohn nodules
	CHEST: Auscultate for murmurs, adventitious lung sounds	Peripheral pulmonary stenosis (PPS) murmur[25]
	ABDOMEN: Palpate for masses, defects, organomegaly Palpate femoral pulses bilaterally	Reducible umbilical hernia; diastasis rectus; cord off
	MSK/NEURO: Perform Ortolani and Barlow maneuvers Assess for symmetric leg length and skin folds Evaluate tone, strength, symmetry of movements	Talipes calcaneovalgus
	REFLEXES: Moro, suck, Babinski, palmar/plantar grasp, stepping, and Galant reflexes	Suck reflex may be hard to elicit, (+) Babinski
	GENITALIA: Labial adhesions (♀) Circumcision status, 2 descended testes (♂)	Testes may appear large for age due to testosterone surge between days 10 and 90[26]
	SKIN: Lesions, rashes, bruising, birthmarks	Seborrheic hyperplasia; milia; hyperpigmented macules of transient neonatal pustular melanosis; seborrheic dermatitis (cradle cap); sucking blisters[24]

YOUR TOOLS	
Screenings:	2nd newborn metabolic screening, if not already done Maternal postpartum depression screening
Immunizations:	None, unless deferred at hospital and newborn visit

<table>
<tr><td rowspan="6">Anticipatory Guidance:</td><td colspan="2">Baby Joys, Baby Blues, and Breastfeeding (the First Month of Life)
Anticipatory guidance at this age centers on the 3 Bs—breast/bottle feeding, breathing, and beds</td></tr>
<tr><td>Nutrition:</td><td>Continue to offer breast milk (or formula) as the sole nutrition source; feed 8–12 times in 24-hour period
Review signs of hunger (hands to face, increased alertness, moving tongue/mouth; crying is a late sign)
Educate mothers on the changes that occur at the breast with continued breastfeeding, such as less engorgement, milk being made on demand with suckling, less letdown sensation
Vitamin D 400 IU daily, if not offering >½ feeds from breast milk
If offering formula, make a fresh bottle with every feeding (1 scoop formula for every 2 oz of water). Encourage paced-bottle feeding, so infant controls flow and intake</td></tr>
<tr><td>Elimination:</td><td>Breastfeeding stools will likely remain frequent and copious until ~6 weeks of age, then the frequency may decrease[17]
Formula-fed infants have brown to tan stools; will likely continue with 1–2/day</td></tr>
<tr><td>Sleep:</td><td>Sleep will continue to be primary activity but should be starting to settle into pattern
SIDS reduction practices should be reviewed (i.e., swaddle, continue to put back to sleep in a crib or co-sleeper, no bed sharing, no secondhand smoke exposure)</td></tr>
<tr><td>Trajectory:</td><td>Growth expectations → Gain about 1 oz/day and can expect a growth spurt at about 6–8 weeks
Upcoming milestones → Increasing periods of wakefulness and periods of crying in the next 2 months, lifting head, cooing, improving neck/head control</td></tr>
<tr><td>Safety:</td><td>Car seat should be a 5-point harness, backward-facing infant carrier in the back seat
No use of infant swings until baby is able to hold neck stable
Review postpartum depression symptoms
Prepare family for increasing episodes of infant crying and discuss techniques to handle. Encourage a safety plan for never shaking a baby. Families should understand that this milestone peaks at ~2 months and then begins to lessen. Crying at this stage is unexpected and unexplainable, may not stop no matter what is done, can appear as though it is painful, can be long-lasting, and occurs more frequently in the afternoons and evenings[27]</td></tr>
</table>

NEWBORNS

WHAT YOU MIGHT HEAR	FOLLOW-UP QUESTIONS	WAYS OF VALIDATING THE CONCERN	EDUCATION YOU CAN PROVIDE & EXAMPLE EDUCATIONAL PHRASE(S)
At the newborn visit: "My baby is not getting enough milk."	• "Tell me more about how the baby is feeding." • "What clues or signals is the baby giving you that tells you your baby is not full?"	"You are right! There is not a lot of milk in these early days and what you are making isn't enough to help the baby grow, but what the body is doing is so important that Mother Nature had the baby store energy during pregnancy to account for this during the first 3 days."	• Importance/role of colostrum • Early milk production physiology • Milk intake in relation to size of infant's stomach and feeding pattern changes as milk "comes in" "Your breast is currently making a highly concentrated form of breast milk called colostrum. It is more like medicine than milk. Like medicine, a little goes a long way, so even just a teaspoon of colostrum is able to coat the entire GI tract and protect it from dangerous viruses and bacteria, while also providing enough antibodies to fight off infections that might get in through other ways. Once the GI tract is safely sealed, your body will start making milk at just the right amounts for the baby's stomach, which is about the size of a walnut right now. Like a gas tank, because it is so small, it can only hold a small amount of milk at one time and it will need to be refilled very frequently."
At the newborn, 2-week, or 1-month visit: "My baby is not good at breastfeeding."	• "Tell me more about why you think he is not good at breastfeeding." • "What do you mean when you say, 'not good at breastfeeding'?"	• "It sounds like you are worried about how he attaches to the breast…" • "Breastfeeding is a learning process for both mom and baby, so it is not unusual to feel clumsy or frustrated with it at times." • "So, when she nurses, it causes you pain, which I am sure makes it feel like you or the baby is doing something wrong…"	• Breastfeeding is often the very first lesson babies learn • Performing a latch assessment • Signs of a good and satisfied feed "Babies aren't necessarily born knowing how to breastfeed efficiently or effectively. Many babies need help to learn how to drink milk from the breast. They have to learn how to pull the milk into their mouth, swallow without choking, and breathe all at the same time. Sometimes it is messy, and it feels awkward." "I would love to have an opportunity to watch you and your little one during a feeding, so that I can show you some tricks that might help you teach baby how to breastfeed without hurting you. Would that be something you would be interested in?"

WHAT YOU MIGHT HEAR	FOLLOW-UP QUESTIONS	WAYS OF VALIDATING THE CONCERN	EDUCATION YOU CAN PROVIDE & EXAMPLE EDUCATIONAL PHRASE(S)
At the 2-week visit: "I think that my breasts might have stopped making milk."	• "What do you mean by your breasts stopped making milk?" • "Tell me more about why you believe your breasts might not be making milk."	• "This whole milk making process is a bit of a rollercoaster, isn't it?" • "I know how unusual it is to one day feel your breasts are full and then suddenly have that sensation stop."	• Milk production physiology changes after 2 weeks • Nursing stimulates milk production • Milk composition changes "Because the breasts can only store so much milk and the baby will eventually need more than the breast can store, after about 2 weeks, the breast actually goes from making and storing milk in the breast, which is what made the breasts feel so heavy and full, to making milk more on demand. When baby nurses, the body starts to produce customized milk, so it goes straight to the baby and no storage is needed." "Since you aren't storing as much milk, that feeling of fullness decreases, but the breast is still making milk, and in fact, is doing a better job customizing the milk for the baby in the moment."
At the 2-week visit or later: "I have to go back to work, so I should just start formula now so he is used to it."	• "Tell me more about your work." • "How have others (in your job or in your family) handled having a new baby and returning to work?" • "What are the challenges you see with breastfeeding and work?"	• "I can see the many challenges you are facing with your return to work." • "It sounds like others in your same situation have struggled to balance work and breastfeeding because of the fast pace at your job." • "I hear you'd want to continue breastfeeding but are feeling like that is an impossible goal."	• Reinforce self-efficacy by using current success as example • Any amount of breast milk is beneficial for the infant, so it doesn't have to be "all or nothing" • Information on state laws "Babies don't want to give up the things they enjoy the most, like nursing and mother's milk, so transitioning to a bottle can be hard. One idea is for day care to give a bottle when you're at work but you continue to nurse when you're at home with the baby. Any time at the breast offers some health benefits." "If you can continue to offer breast milk to the baby by having the time and a space for pumping at work, the baby's risk of illness is lower, which means fewer missed days from work. It is a win–win for everyone."

NEWBORNS

WHAT YOU MIGHT HEAR	FOLLOW-UP QUESTIONS	WAYS OF VALIDATING THE CONCERN	EDUCATION YOU CAN PROVIDE & EXAMPLE EDUCATIONAL PHRASE(S)
At any visit from 2 months on: "When I am at work and I am pumping, I can't make enough milk to keep up with his daily appetite."	• "Tell me about a typical day at work and your pumping routine." • "How is the caregiver feeding your son when using your breast milk?"	• "It can be challenging to keep up with your baby's rapid growth when pumping at work." • "I hear that you are worried that you may have to supplement your baby or possibly stop breastfeeding if you don't make enough milk each day, but there are many different combinations and ways to nourish your baby."	• How caregivers can use paced bottle feeding to more closely mimic breastfeeding • Power pumping trial to see if it increases production • Milk storage "We can try some techniques to increase the amount of milk you pump, but the most important message I want to share with you is that any breast milk you give to your baby is a lifelong gift, and no matter if we have to add some bows and ribbons to that gift in the form of a supplement, it doesn't change the fact that he is getting a gift every day."
At the 4-month visit: "I think my milk must taste bad or she is ready for other types of foods because she is refusing to nurse."	• "Tell me more about what she does when she refuses to nurse." • "What cues make you think that the milk flavor has changed?" • "How long has it been that she is not wanting to nurse?"	• "It sounds like you're concerned that your baby is starting to wean; however, self-weaning is rare before the first birthday, so it may be a case of something else distracting her from nursing, like an infection." • "It can be upsetting not knowing why something that was going well suddenly changes."	• Baby-led weaning rarely occurs before the end of the first year • Why and when nursing strikes occur (developmentally and emotionally challenging times) • Developmentally distractable ages can make nursing more difficult for some infants • Importance of continuing to empty breasts and feeding baby "It is not uncommon for babies to go on strike from nursing when there is something physical, developmental, or emotional happening in their worlds. It may just be your baby's way of asking us to look a little deeper to make sure that there isn't something causing her pain, distress, or disruption." "Babies are a lot like us adults, they have a lot going on in their heads and a lot that they are trying to work on. If they are stressed, they may not want to eat a home-cooked meal but rather do fast food so that they can get back to the task at hand."

WHAT YOU MIGHT HEAR	FOLLOW-UP QUESTIONS	WAYS OF VALIDATING THE CONCERN	EDUCATION YOU CAN PROVIDE & EXAMPLE EDUCATIONAL PHRASE(S)
At the 4- or 6-month visit: "He must be upset with me because he always bites my nipple when feeding."	• "What makes you think that he might be doing this on purpose?" • "Does he have teeth yet?" • "Does he act like he might be teething?" • "Tell me about how you and he react when he bites during a feeding."	• "It sounds like it is upsetting when he bites during a feeding for both you and him." • "I can definitely understand why you would be concerned about this, as it could impact how you two move forward around breastfeeding."	• Teething may be the underlying culprit • Infants don't understand the concept of intentional harm • Many times, infants are practicing their tongue movements in preparation for solids and bite accidentally "This is a very common concern at this age. It can be due to sore and swollen gums or he could be practicing tongue movements in preparation for starting solid foods. When the tongue is not covering that lower gumline, he can certainly pinch your nipple between his gums or his erupting teeth! It's best to end the feeding by putting your finger in between the gums to break the suction, while calmly telling him, 'No biting!' He'll quickly begin to understand playing with his food is not a great idea, if he wants to be able to continue enjoyable nursing times." "While it may feel very personal, as it is your nipple he is biting down on, remember that babies don't understand or have the capacity to inflict intentional harm. He likely just moves his tongue back when he finishes eating and forgets. You can watch for this and remove him from the breast to avoid future incidents."
At any well visit: "My friends are all telling me that I am spoiling him when I let him nurse whenever he wants."	• "How do you feel about having him nurse when he signals he needs it?" • "Do you think he is wanting something other than food or love when he feeds?"	• "It sounds like you are questioning whether you are interpreting and responding to his needs appropriately." • "I hear you and your friends may have different ways of caring for your infants and that is OK. There is no absolutely 'right' way to do this parenting thing."	• Benefits of secure attachment are far reaching and set the child up for strong social–emotional bonds in the future • Nutritive and nonnutritive benefits to sucking "Parenting is one of the hardest jobs we take on in our lives and it doesn't come with a manual, but mother's intuition is real, so if you respond to his needs by putting him to the breast, you are actually not spoiling him, but showing him that he is loved and that he can trust you to take care of him when he needs something."

NUTRITION

NATURAL FOODS:	Exclusive breastfeeding recommended; iron-fortified formula is alternative • Breastfeeding: 6–10×/day using on-demand cues; 10 minutes per side of active feeding • Bottle feeding: 6–8 feeds/day; 3–4 oz q3–4 hours (average 26–32 oz)[28] No other liquids/fluids needed (including water)
VITAMINS:	Vitamin D (400 IU) daily if breastfeeding; vitamin B_{12} if breastfeeding mother is vegan and doesn't take a B_{12} supplement Prenatal vitamins for breastfeeding mother, as anemia in mother can reduce milk supply
IRON SOURCES:	Iron found in breast milk (lactoferrin) is highly bioavailable, so no supplement is needed for term infants[28] Use iron-fortified formula if supplementing or not breastfeeding
GRAINS:	Mostly useful for the maternal diet at this age
ADDED SUGAR/SALT:	No additives should be put into pumped breast milk or formula
TEETH:	Oral health care for mother is important for preventing early childhood caries in child later in life, so encourage routine dental care for mother
DAIRY:	Breast milk or formula

ELIMINATION

URINATION:	6–8 wet diapers/day	
STOOLING:	Breastfed: Yellow, loose, seedy; may be irregular and infrequent	Formula fed: Tan to brown; 3–4/day

SLEEP

POSITION:	Put on back for sleeping
QUANTITY:	4–5 hours/night; 2–3 naps; total: 12–16 hours
ROUTINE:	Routine around sleep may or may not be emerging at this time More frequent nighttime awakenings for breastfed babies Pacifier use OK for sleep and to reduce risk of SIDS but should not be used throughout day[18]
SLEEP SITE & SAFETY:	Co-sleeper or crib with room sharing; no bed sharing[18] Snug mattress and narrow crib slats in crib No bottles, plush toys, blankets, pillows, bumpers in sleeping area

TRACKING

GROWTH:	Gain 20–30 g/day; typically up 2–2.5 pounds from 2 week visit[10] Should be starting to see some trends with length, weight, HC, and weight-for-length ratio

FAMILY

Family, Including Siblings & Outside Supports:	Division of responsibility Parental time with each other Parental time with other children (without infant)
	Ask about support networks (e.g., mom–baby groups) If not asked previously, discuss family's childcare decisions
Adjustment to Age or Stage:	Screen for maternal depression and sleep Increasing interaction and play with infant
Monetary:	Good time to ask again about food (or formula) insecurity Refer to WIC for assistance, if needed and qualify
Safety:	Creating a safety plan for handling a colicky or crying infant Discuss or screen for caregiver substance use Ask about secondhand smoke, vaping, THC exposure

LEARNING

Physical Development

Gross Motor:	Lifting head up Pushing up in prone	**Fine Motor:**	Grasping objects Bringing hands to midline/mouth

Communication/Language Development

Verbal:	Coos	**Nonverbal:**	Differentiation of cry

Cognitive/Intellectual Development

Intelligence:	None to note	**Problem-Solving:**	Indicates boredom with crying/fussiness

Social–Emotional Development

Connection:	Social smile Responds to caregiver's voice Follows parent's face	**Self-Regulation:**	Hands to mouth

YOUR TOOLS

YOUR INTERVIEW:	*What is your baby doing right now that you are enjoying the most?* *How are you handling the crying milestone?* *Tell me about your sleep schedule.* *Tell me about how breastfeeding is going.*
YOUR OBSERVATIONS:	The infant should be showing increasing responsiveness to caregiver's voice, smile, cuddling, and cooing. A connected caregiver is constantly playing with the infant, stimulating his nervous system and helps develop head and neck control and motor skills. Make note of signs of potential caregiver postpartum depression, as this can greatly impact growth and development.

PHYSICAL EXAM:	COMPLETE PHYSICAL EXAM WITH A SPECIFIC FOCUS ON	NORMAL FINDINGS YOU MIGHT SEE AT THIS AGE
HEAD:	Palpate fontanelles Evaluate for positional skull deformities	Posterior fontanelle typically closed; anterior fontanelle averages 2 cm (2 finger widths)[21]
EYES:	Note red reflexes Assess tracking, ocular mobility, alignment	*Intermittent* strabismic deviations Horizontal (but not across midline) tracking[29]
EARS:	Inspect external ear and tragus for placement, pits, or tags	
NECK:	Assess for full ROM and torticollis	Mild head lag
MOUTH:	Inspect uvula, palate, and gums	Hands to mouth
CHEST:	Auscultate for murmurs, adventitious lung sounds	S3 heart sound; PPS murmur (esp. if premature)
ABDOMEN:	Palpate for masses, wall defects, organomegaly Palpate femoral pulses bilaterally	Diastasis rectus may still be present
MSK/NEURO:	Perform Ortolani and Barlow maneuvers Assess for symmetric leg length and leg skin folds Evaluate tone, strength, symmetry of movements	
REFLEXES:	Moro, suck, rooting, Babinski, palmar/plantar grasp, Galant	Strong palmar and plantar reflex; rooting reflex likely gone
GENITALIA:	Labial adhesions (♀) Circumcision status, 2 descended testes (♂)	Large appearing testes due to testosterone surge between 10 days and 3 months[26]
SKIN:	Lesions, rashes, bruising, birthmarks	Neonatal acne; seborrheic dermatitis (cradle cap); hyperpigmented macules of transient neonatal pustular melanosis[24]

NEWBORNS

	YOUR TOOLS	
SCREENINGS:	Maternal postpartum depression screening	*Optional based on history/risks/practice preference* Developmental screening
IMMUNIZATIONS:	HepB #2 Hib #1 IPV #1 PCV13 #1 DTaP #1 RV #1	

ANTICIPATORY GUIDANCE:

Contentment, Crying, and Connection (2 Months)
The anticipatory guidance at this stage centers on these 4 Cs—crying (both infant and mom), co-sleeping, core strength, and cooing

NUTRITION:	Continue to offer breast milk (or formula) as the primary nutrition source Prescribe vitamin D for exclusively breastfed infants, if not currently using
ELIMINATION:	Breastfeeding stools will continue to be yellow, soft, and almost liquid Remind families that breastfeeding babies may not stool for up to a week at a time
SLEEP:	Baby should be laid in bed before falling asleep so she can learn to self-quiet and put herself to sleep Continue to put back to sleep in a co-sleeper or crib with an emphasis on no bed sharing Emphasize need for routine around sleep
TRAJECTORY:	Growth expectations → Gain about ½ lb/month until 6 months Upcoming milestones → Increasing "tummy time" promotes core strength, rolling front to back, reaching for objects; cooing and infant interactions will lead to babbling, smiling
SAFETY:	Avoid passive smoke exposure Turn hot water heater to <120° Sun safety should be discussed, if seasonally appropriate Car seat should be a 5-point harness, backward-facing infant carrier that is placed in the back seat Review postpartum depression symptoms and provide resources for the family Discuss and prepare families for continued episodes of unexplainable infant crying and provide techniques to handle

2 Months

NUTRITION

Natural Foods:	Exclusive breastfeeding recommended; iron-fortified formula is alternative • Breastfeeding: 6–10×/day with more routine feedings; easily distractable, so may need a low-stimuli environment for feeds • Bottle feeding: 6–8 feeds/day; 30–32 oz/day Hold complementary foods until 6 months if breastfeeding
Vitamins:	Vitamin D (400 IU) daily if breastfeeding Need iron supplementation for breastfeeding infants at 1 mg/kg/day[28]
Iron Sources:	Iron stores reach lowest nadir at 4–6 months; breast milk low in iron (despite high bioavailability), so for some infants intake is unable to meet demands → AAP recommends supplementing until complementary foods are introduced[28] Use iron-fortified formula if supplementing or not breastfeeding
Grains:	Single-grain (usually rice) cereal OK as first food, if developmentally ready Mix 1 teaspoon cereal with water or formula for a thin consistency and feed with a spoon 1–2× a day; do not offer in a bottle
Added Sugar/Salt:	Avoid added sugar/salts in diet with addition of complementary foods; no honey under the age of 1 year
Teeth:	Hands to mouth and drooling, but no tooth eruption typical
Dairy:	Breast milk or formula

ELIMINATION

Urination:	6–8 wet diapers/day	
Stooling:	Breastfed: Yellow, loose, seedy; may be irregular and infrequent	Formula fed: Tan to brown; 3–4/day

SLEEP

Position:	Put on back for sleeping; stop swaddling when infant begins rolling
Quantity:	4–5 hours/night; 2–4 naps; total: 12–16 hours Sleep stretches should be longer each night
Routine:	Ask about bedtime routine to ensure that this is starting to become a habit More frequent nighttime awakenings for breastfed babies Pacifier use OK for sleep and calming but should not be used throughout day
Sleep Site & Safety:	AAP recommends co-sleeper or crib with room sharing, but no bed sharing Snug mattress and narrow crib slats in crib and no bottles, plush toys, blankets, pillows, bumpers in sleeping area

TRACKING

Growth:	Infant should be beginning to settle into a growth trajectory, with expected gain of about ½ lb per week or 2 lb per month Infant usually has doubled birth weight

FAMILY

FAMILY, INCLUDING SIBLINGS & OUTSIDE SUPPORTS:	Division of responsibility Parental time with each other; parental time with other children (without infant) Inquire about sibling jealousy
	Changes in support networks (e.g., mom–baby groups) If not previously discussed, family's childcare decisions, if parent(s) returning to work, or respite resources, if staying at home
ADJUSTMENT TO AGE OR STAGE:	Ask about infant temperament How is family handling a crying infant
MONEY:	Inquire about food, housing, utility, or employment insecurity Ensure the family is using government nutritional assistance programs, if needed and qualify
SAFETY:	Discuss sibling safety, if older children in the house Ask about how parents/caregivers handle differences in parenting styles/philosophies/strategies Ask about secondhand smoke, vaping, THC exposure

LEARNING

PHYSICAL DEVELOPMENT

GROSS MOTOR:	Good head control Pushes up on elbows Sits with support Rolling from front to back	**FINE MOTOR:**	Reaching for objects Bats at objects Brings hands together in clapping motion

COMMUNICATION/LANGUAGE DEVELOPMENT

VERBAL:	Babbles more expressively and spontaneously Imitates sounds	**NONVERBAL:**	Clearer behavior to indicate needs

COGNITIVE/INTELLECTUAL DEVELOPMENT

INTELLIGENCE:	Responds to changes in environment	**PROBLEM-SOLVING:**	Indicates boredom with crying/fussiness

SOCIAL–EMOTIONAL DEVELOPMENT

CONNECTION:	Smiles spontaneously Responds to affection Social cough Laugh and squeal begin Indicates pleasure/displeasure	**SELF-REGULATION:**	Solidified self-consoling skills

YOUR TOOLS	
YOUR INTERVIEW:	*Tell me about how breastfeeding is going. How is breastfeeding different now from the last time we saw you?* *What is your plan for introducing table foods/solids? Is the infant beginning to show interest in family foods?* *Tell me about your sleep schedule.* *What is your baby doing right now that you are enjoying the most? What is the most difficult thing that your baby does right now?*
YOUR OBSERVATIONS:	The infant is not usually sitting just yet but rolling from tummy to back is a distinct possibility. If you put the baby prone on the exam table, she may fuss and cry, but with a little help she'll likely roll onto her back, as the white exam paper is not nearly as interesting as the faces of her family. There may be smiling, laughing, and squealing, and responding to changes in the caregiver's expressions. It continues to be important to assess for signs of postpartum depression.

PHYSICAL EXAM:		COMPLETE PHYSICAL EXAM WITH A SPECIFIC FOCUS ON	NORMAL FINDINGS YOU MIGHT SEE AT THIS AGE
	HEAD:	Palpate fontanelles Evaluate for positional skull deformities	Posterior fontanelle typically closed; anterior fontanelle with variable size, but still open; friction alopecia; mild plagiocephaly
	EYES:	Note red reflexes Assess tracking, ocular mobility, alignment (corneal light reflex, cover–uncover test)	Conjugate gaze appreciated on ocular mobility Vertical and circular eye movements Visual convergence
	NECK:	Assess for full ROM and torticollis	Mild to no head lag
	MOUTH:	Inspect uvula, palate, and gums	Lots of drooling
	CHEST:	Auscultate for murmurs, adventitious lung sounds	S3 heart sound
	ABDOMEN:	Palpate for masses, organomegaly Palpate femoral pulses bilaterally	
	MSK/NEURO:	Perform Ortolani and Barlow maneuvers Assess for symmetric leg length and leg skin folds Evaluate tone, strength, symmetry of movements	
	REFLEXES:	Palmar, Babinski, ATNR, Gallant, Landau, STNR, and TLR	Moro, stepping, and suck reflexes have disappeared
	GENITALIA:	Labial adhesions (♀) Circumcision status, 2 descended testes (♂)	Retractile testes[26]
	SKIN:	Lesions, rashes, bruising, birthmarks	Neonatal acne; seborrheic dermatitis (cradle cap), drool rash on chin, neck, and/or upper chest

<table>
<tr><td rowspan="10" style="writing-mode:vertical-lr">INFANTS</td><td colspan="3" align="center">**YOUR TOOLS**</td><td rowspan="10" style="writing-mode:vertical-lr">4 Months</td></tr>
<tr><td>**SCREENINGS:**</td><td colspan="2">Maternal postpartum depression screening
Risk assessment for iron deficiency anemia, especially if exclusively breastfeeding</td><td>*Optional based on history/risks/practice preference*
Developmental screening</td></tr>
</table>

	YOUR TOOLS		
SCREENINGS:	Maternal postpartum depression screening Risk assessment for iron deficiency anemia, especially if exclusively breastfeeding		*Optional based on history/risks/practice preference* Developmental screening
IMMUNIZATIONS:	IPV #2 DTaP #2 Hib #2	PCV13 #2 RV #2 HepB* #3	
ANTICIPATORY GUIDANCE:			

Contentment, Crying, and Connections (4 Months)

The anticipatory guidance at this stage centers on these 3 Cs—continue primary nutrition, complementary foods (when to introduce), and being conscientious (reminding parents to be mindful of infant's new mobility)

NUTRITION:	Continue to offer breast milk (or formula) as the primary nutrition source and wait to introduce solids until the child is developmentally ready May begin complementary foods once tongue thrust has disappeared and infant can sit without support (usually closer to 6 months) Increasing demands for breastfeeds for several days without satisfaction may signal readiness for solids Recommend that first food be an iron-fortified single-grain cereal or red meat. Start with 1 teaspoon and then increase to 1 tablespoon as accepted
ELIMINATION:	Stooling may change with addition of complementary foods
SLEEP:	Begin weaning nighttime feeds Continue to put back to sleep in a co-sleeper or crib with no bed sharing
TRAJECTORY:	Growth expectations → Gain about 2 lb/month until 6 months Upcoming milestones → Rolling back to front, object transfer, grasping toys with hand, more engagement, and more peek-a-boo play
SAFETY:	Avoid passive smoke exposure Review safe use of medications (e.g., dose by weight, use dropper or cup that comes with the medication, no ibuprofen until at least 6 months, etc.) Review that infant crying will continue but will be decreasing in intensity and frequency and remind parents about some of the techniques to handle these episodes Rolling and increased mobility increase fall risk. Parents need to keep one hand on baby at all times

*Depends on immunization series used

NUTRITION

NATURAL FOODS:	Continued breastfeeding recommended; iron-fortified formula is alternative • Breastfeeding: 6–10×/day with more routine feedings • Bottle feeding: 6–8 feeds/day; 30–32 oz/day Complementary first foods (after cereals) can be any single ingredient foods, but typically green vegetables or non-citrus fruits offered in a puree. Offer 1–2 oz of water in a cup with complementary foods to practice cup use skills
VITAMINS:	Vitamin D (400 IU) daily if breastfeeding and prenatal vitamins for breastfeeding mother AAP notes parents can stop iron supplements for breastfed infants once they are eating complementary foods 2–3 times a day[30]
IRON SOURCES:	Complementary foods can be iron-fortified, but some complementary foods higher in iron include green peas, sweet potatoes, squash, meats (red meat, liver, poultry), prunes, and apricots[31,32]
GRAINS:	Single-grain cereals (rice or wheat) common; mix with water, formula or breast milk for a thin consistency. Recommend offering after breast or bottle feeds; expect infant will eat only a few baby spoonfuls at the main family meal
ADDED SUGAR/SALT:	No honey until 1 year of age. No added sugar or salt in diet and avoid canned/processed foods as base for purees
TEETH:	First teeth tend to begin to erupt now, starting with the lower central incisors; fluoride varnish should be applied every 3–6 months from tooth eruption until the child is established with a dental home[33]
DAIRY:	Breast milk or formula; avoid animal or nut milks due to risk of microscopic enterocolitis and electrolyte/fluid shifts[34]

ELIMINATION

URINATION:	6–8 wet diapers/day	
STOOLING:	Breastfed: Becomes more odiferous with addition of solid foods; tan to brown; more frequency than 2- and 4-month patterns	Formula fed: Tan to brown; 1–3/day

SLEEP

POSITION:	Put on back for sleeping; stop swaddling as normally able to roll
QUANTITY:	5–8 hours/night; 2–3 naps; total: 12–16 hours "Sleeping through the night"—a 5-hour stretch qualifies[35]
ROUTINE:	Should now have a routine; may include bath, cleaning teeth/gums, reading a story prior to bedtime May want to begin weaning pacifier use after 6 months; should not use throughout day[36]
SLEEP SITE & SAFETY:	AAP recommends co-sleeper or crib with room sharing, but no bed sharing Snug mattress and narrow crib slats in crib; no bottles, plush toys, blankets, pillows, bumpers in sleeping area

TRACKING

GROWTH:	Weight gains slow after 6 months; typically very chubby at this age

FAMILY

Family, Including Siblings & Outside Supports:	Typically clearer role definitions within the family Sibling safety should be discussed, especially if siblings are helping with care of infant
	Some of the early supports begin to fade, but there is increased demand on time from infant Caregiver(s) may need respite time Discuss outside support if parent/caregivers are returning to work
Adjustment to Age or Stage:	Ask about interactive activities with infant Increasing mobility
Money:	Returning to work/childcare decisions
Safety:	Day care provider and licensing/accreditation Infant CPR training Ask about secondhand smoke, vaping, THC exposure

LEARNING

Physical Development

Gross Motor:	Sits with minimal support Rolling back to front	**Fine Motor:**	Holds blocks/toys with 2 hands Object transfer

Communication/Language Development

Verbal:	Single consonant vocalizations (ah, eh, oh) Vocal turn taking	**Nonverbal:**	Points with index finger Smiles responsively

Cognitive/Intellectual Development

Intelligence:	Recognizes own name Turns toward sounds	**Problem-Solving:**	Removes blanket from face Shakes toys

Social–Emotional Development

Connection:	Interacts with parents/caregivers and fears unfamiliar people Tries to talk to an image in the mirror	**Self-Regulation:**	Holds toy to comfort self Puts things in mouth for calming

YOUR TOOLS		
YOUR INTERVIEW:	*How will you introduce solids like cereal, meats, fruits, and vegetables? Tell me about how the introduction of solids is going.* *How do you feel about transitioning to providing fluids in a cup?* *What is your baby doing right now that you are enjoying the most?* *What is the most difficult thing that your baby does right now?*	
YOUR OBSERVATIONS:	Continued infant–parent attachment, but some increased mobility, entertaining self with infant toys, playing with hands and feet and initiating games like peek-a-boo helps the 6-month-old begin to gain self-efficacy. Great interest in the surrounding world and loves the sound of crinkling exam paper.	
PHYSICAL EXAM:	**COMPLETE PHYSICAL EXAM WITH A SPECIFIC FOCUS ON**	**NORMAL FINDINGS YOU MIGHT SEE AT THIS AGE**
	HEAD: Palpate fontanelles Evaluate for positional skull deformities	Anterior fontanelle with variable size (3–6 cm), typically still open (3% of infants closed at 6 months)[21]; friction alopecia; mild plagiocephaly
	EYES: Note red reflexes Assess tracking, ocular mobility, alignment	Following past midline Recognizing favorite toy from a distance[29]
	NECK: Assess for full ROM and torticollis	No head lag
	MOUTH: Inspect uvula, palate, and gums	Eruption of first primary tooth/teeth (usually lower first incisor)[37] Palatine tonsils
	CHEST: Auscultate for murmurs, adventitious lung sounds	PPS murmur[25]
	ABDOMEN: Palpate for masses, HSM Palpate femoral pulses bilaterally	
	MSK/NEURO: Perform Ortolani and Barlow maneuvers Assess for symmetric leg length and skin folds Evaluate tone, strength, symmetry of movements	Sitting without support or sitting with one-handed support Joint attention with caregiver possible
	REFLEXES: Palmar, Babinski, ATNR, Gallant, Landau, STNR, and TLR	Plantar, Babinski, and Gallant reflexes remain
	GENITALIA: Labial adhesions (♀) Circumcision status, 2 descended testes (♂)	Retractile testes

YOUR TOOLS	
Screenings: Maternal postpartum depression screening Oral health risk assessment	*Optional based on history/risks/practice preference* Lead toxicity risk assessment Developmental screening

Immunizations:	HepB #3 IPV #3 DTaP #3 PCV13 #3	Hib* #3 RV* #3 Influenza (2 doses separated by 1 month), if seasonally appropriate

Anticipatory Guidance:		
	Contentment, Crying, and Connections (6 Months) The anticipatory guidance at this stage centers on these 3 Cs—changes in stools, complementary foods (how to introduce more), and coming milestone of crawling (begin baby proofing the house)	
	Nutrition:	Continue to offer breast milk (or formula) as primary nutrition source and complementary foods after May begin complementary foods once tongue thrust has disappeared and can sit without support Complementary foods should serve as a bonding experience between infant and adult, is a time to practice fine motor skills, and should be fun and enjoyable. Families should not stress if the child only eats a small amount, is not interested in the foods, or the majority ends up on the floor, in his hair, or anywhere but in his mouth Introduce new pureed food every 2–4 days and watch for potential signs of food allergies (e.g., hives, flushing, coughing/wheezing, vomiting/diarrhea, difficulty breathing, etc.) Avoid honey until 1 year of age (due to infant botulism risk)
	Elimination:	Stooling may change with addition of complementary foods
	Sleep:	Begin weaning nighttime feeds Continue to put back to sleep in a crib and continue to discourage bed sharing
	Trajectory:	Growth expectations → Growth trajectory to slow between 6 and 12 months Upcoming milestones → Pulling to a stand and crawling, using fingers to feed self, begins repeating single consonant sounds, increased stranger apprehension
	Safety:	Avoid passive smoke exposure Car seat should be a 5-point harness, backward-facing infant carrier that is located in the back seat Postpartum depression symptoms may appear with return to work or decrease in social supports, so review Increased mobility will lead to curious yet unstable babies, so it is time to begin babyproofing the house with gates, cabinet locks, and corner covers

*Depends on immunization series used

NUTRITION	
Natural Foods:	Solids usually offered as 3 meals per day with 3 snacks a day Offer new foods as snacks and established foods as meals Increased self-feeding with finger foods No spill cup with water (no juice) Offer solids when in a high chair and milk or formula when in caregiver's arms • Breastfeeding: 4–5×/day • Bottle feeding: 3–4 feeds/day; 16–24 oz/day
Vitamins:	Continue with vitamin D supplementation if breastfeeding infant is receiving <1 liter of supplemental formula per day[28]
Iron Sources:	1–2 oz of pureed red meat; 1 oz of iron-fortified cereal meets daily requirement (usually divided into 2 servings a day); serve with foods high in vitamin C for better absorption (orange, grapefruit, kiwi, strawberries, broccoli, tomatoes, and peppers)
Grains:	Continue grain cereals, but whole-grain, cooked pasta and Cheerios are good sources as well
Added Sugar/Salt:	Avoid sugar-sweetened beverages, so most juices not recommended[38]
Teeth:	Usually has 2–4 teeth (lower and/or upper central incisors);[37] brushing with smear (about the size of a grain of rice) of fluoride toothpaste and soft toothbrush twice a day recommended[39,40]
Dairy:	Breast milk or formula is still recommended
ELIMINATION	
Urination:	8–12 wet diapers/day
Stooling:	Usually less frequent than before due to slower gastrointestinal transit time
SLEEP	
Position:	Continue to put back to sleep, but decreased SIDS risk
Quantity:	6–7 hours/night; 2–3 naps; total: 12–16 hours Sleep stretches should be longer each night but may also see increased nighttime awakenings
Routine:	Baby should be laid in bed before falling asleep so she can learn to self-quiet and put herself to sleep Pacifier use OK for sleep or calming but ideally should not be used at other times of day
Sleep Site & Safety:	Most have moved to a crib, if previously in a bassinet or co-sleeper, and may be out of parent's room Put mattress on lowest level and always put sides up in the crib, as standing up in crib becomes common
TRACKING	
Growth:	Growth slows after 6 months, but still gaining about ½ pound a month[10]

INFANTS

FAMILY		
FAMILY, INCLUDING SIBLINGS & OUTSIDE SUPPORTS:	Ask about marriage and date nights for parents Sibling involvement with a reminder to parents to never leave infant alone with sibling Caregivers outside of the parents and ensure they are also following same feeding, sleep, and discipline plans	
ADJUSTMENT TO AGE OR STAGE:	How is the family responding to the child's emotional development (e.g., stranger apprehension and separation anxiety)? Emotional development including frustration, anger, and fear	
MONEY:	Discuss food insecurity or worry about having enough money to buy formula (refer to WIC or SNAP benefits, if eligible) Inquire about financial support	
SAFETY:	Ask about marital problems/relationship problems for the caregivers Discuss plans for discipline and potentially how the caregiver was parented/disciplined Ask about secondhand smoke, vaping, THC exposure	

LEARNING			
PHYSICAL DEVELOPMENT			
GROSS MOTOR:	Crawling Pulling to a stand	**FINE MOTOR:**	Pincer grasp Likes to shake, bang, throw, and drop objects
COMMUNICATION/LANGUAGE DEVELOPMENT			
VERBAL:	Repetitive consonants and vowels (e.g., "ma-ma," "da-da," "be-be") Understands "no"	**NONVERBAL:**	Points objects out
COGNITIVE/INTELLECTUAL DEVELOPMENT			
INTELLIGENCE:	Object permanence	**PROBLEM-SOLVING:**	Likes cause-and-effect toys (drop and dump)
SOCIAL–EMOTIONAL DEVELOPMENT			
CONNECTION:	Stranger apprehension Plays peek-a-boo and so-big games	**SELF-REGULATION:**	Seeks parents for comfort and as a resource May use a transitional object

YOUR TOOLS	
YOUR INTERVIEW:	*How is feeding time at your home? What questions do you have about solids, family foods? What trends have you noted in terms of the amount of breast milk or formula the infant is taking? How is your breast milk supply?* *How do you know when your baby is hungry and when your baby is full?* *What is your baby doing right now that you are enjoying the most?* *What is the most difficult thing that your baby does right now?*
YOUR OBSERVATIONS:	A new found sense of mobility and dexterity have the 9-month-old pulling to a stand and potentially cruising around the exam room ready to grab the smallest bit of lint or paper with the increasingly improved pincer grasp. A growing awareness of object permanence may have her looking for toy hidden under a transitional object (like a blanket) or she may be too apprehensive of strangers to want to play much, which may make for a bit more difficult of an exam.

PHYSICAL EXAM:	COMPLETE PHYSICAL EXAM WITH A SPECIFIC FOCUS ON		NORMAL FINDINGS YOU MIGHT SEE AT THIS AGE
	HEAD:	Palpate fontanelles	Anterior fontanelle with variable size, but still open for 80% of infants
	EYES:	Note red reflexes Assess tracking, ocular mobility, alignment (corneal light reflex, cover–uncover test)	
	NECK:	Assess for ROM and lymphadenopathy	
	MOUTH:	Inspect uvula, palate, and gums	2–4 teeth (usually upper and lower 1st incisors); palatine tonsils
	CHEST:	Auscultate for murmurs, adventitious lung sounds	S3 and S4
	ABDOMEN:	Palpate for masses, organomegaly Palpate femoral pulses bilaterally	
	MSK/NEURO:	Perform Ortolani and Barlow maneuvers Evaluate tone, strength, and symmetry of movements Assess for joint attention (eye contact and nonverbal or verbal affective response)	
	REFLEXES:	Plantar, Babinski, parachute	Parachute reflex appears
	GENITALIA:	Labial adhesions (♀) Circumcision status, 2 descended testes (♂)	Retractile testes

YOUR TOOLS		
SCREENINGS:	Developmental screening Oral health risk assessment	*Optional based on history/risks/practice preference* Postpartum depression screening Lead toxicity risk assessment
IMMUNIZATIONS:	Typically none unless catch-up immunizations are required	
ANTICIPATORY GUIDANCE:	**Determination, Drooling, and Da-Da (9 Months)** Anticipatory guidance at this stage centers on these 3 Ds—diet, drooling, and dental home	
	NUTRITION:	Continue to offer breast milk (or formula) in conjunction with expanding diet of complementary foods Continue iron-fortified foods and plan to transition to whole (4%) cow's milk at 1 year Avoid honey until 1 year of age (due to infant botulism risk) Portion sizes for age are 1 teaspoon of each food group at each meal, plus 2–3 high carbohydrate snacks Offer new foods for snacks, understanding that it may take up to 10–15 attempts for an infant to accept a new food, texture, or flavor Drooling is a harbinger of erupting teeth, so discuss cleaning teeth daily • Clean teeth with soft bristled toothbrush and a smear of toothpaste twice a day • Offer safe teething remedies (use cold washcloth, but avoid frozen teething rings, numbing gel, etc.) Emphasize the importance of establishing with a dental home by the time the child is 1 year of age
	ELIMINATION:	Stooling patterns may change with addition of complementary foods
	SLEEP:	Lower the mattress on the crib, as standing and climbing is common Encourage routines around sleep
	TRAJECTORY:	Early literacy and book resources can change trajectory of infant's school success Upcoming milestones → Cruising, jabbering, separation anxiety, and 1–3 words in vocabulary
	SAFETY:	Continue to keep baby in a rear-facing car seat in the back seat until 2 years old, or whenever child reaches weight or height limit for car seat Discuss water safety and the need to supervise children near any water sources (e.g., toilets, dog water bowls, and during baths) Encourage families to consider taking an infant CPR course, if they have not done so already

INFANTS

9 Months

NUTRITION

NATURAL FOODS:	Encourage continued breastfeeding, if mutually desirable Eating less than previously (may eat 1 large meal, 2 smaller meals, and 2–3 snacks) Wide variety of foods, including fruits and veggies, should be offered Food struggles common Snacks should be rich in complex carbohydrates, but minimal sweets Like finger foods but are messy eaters
VITAMINS:	Vitamin D–fortified whole milk Other vitamin supplements are not necessary, if eating balanced diet
IRON SOURCES:	Limit milk intake to ≤24 oz, as milk can bind iron Continue iron-fortified cereal or meats with vitamin C–containing foods to improve absorption
GRAINS:	Single-grain baby cereals, finger foods (whole wheat pasta, Cheerios, crackers)
ADDED SUGAR/SALT:	Avoid added salts and sugars, such as sugar-sweetened beverages and juices
TEETH:	Now with 4–8 teeth; parents should be brushing teeth with a smear of fluoridated toothpaste twice a day
DAIRY:	Transition bottle-fed formula feeders to whole milk in a cup. If weaning or only nursing a few times a day/night, transition to whole milk in a cup at 2–3 cups (480–720 mL)

ELIMINATION

URINATION:	8–12 wet diapers/day
STOOLING:	Unchanged from previous visits

SLEEP

POSITION:	Put on back for sleeping
QUANTITY:	6–8 hours/night; 1–2 naps of 1–3 hours each; total: 11–14 hours Sleep stretches should be longer at night
ROUTINE:	Routine should include bedtime story/reading and toothbrushing Encouraging a strict routine can help set boundaries for toddlers
SLEEP SITE & SAFETY:	Usually still in a crib May be able to crawl out of crib, even if mattress on lowest setting

TRACKING

GROWTH:	Typically have tripled birth weight and doubled birth length

FAMILY

FAMILY, INCLUDING SIBLINGS & OUTSIDE SUPPORTS:	Inquire about whether the caregivers' relationships are doing OK and see if they are creating time for "date nights" Ask about role of sibling in caring for infant and emphasize the need to never leave infant alone with a sibling Outside day care or in-home day care
ADJUSTMENT TO AGE OR STAGE:	How is the family handling the increased mobility? Attachment to parents and separation anxiety
MONEY:	Ensure that the child has ongoing health insurance, as may need to re-enroll in some plans after the first birthday Ask about what types of activities the family does with the child that don't require money and suggest things like story time at the local library, playing at a park, etc.
SAFETY:	Environmental hazards in the home or neighborhood now that the infant is more mobile (e.g., second floor apartment, living near high traffic area, noise or air pollution, etc.) Question secondhand smoke, vaping, THC exposure in both the home and in the car

LEARNING

PHYSICAL DEVELOPMENT

GROSS MOTOR:	Stands alone Cruises Takes a few steps alone	**FINE MOTOR:**	Puts items into and takes them out of containers

COMMUNICATION/LANGUAGE DEVELOPMENT

VERBAL:	Jabbers with inflection of normal speech 1–3 words in vocabulary in addition to ma-ma and da-da	**NONVERBAL:**	Protoimperative pointing (pointing to object of interest)

COGNITIVE/INTELLECTUAL DEVELOPMENT

INTELLIGENCE:	Understands one command with a gesture Identifies a person on request (e.g., "Where is daddy?")	**PROBLEM-SOLVING:**	Looks for a dropped or hidden object

SOCIAL–EMOTIONAL DEVELOPMENT

CONNECTION:	Plays peek-a-boo and pat-a-cake Waves bye-bye Strong attachment to parent, which leads to separation anxiety	**SELF-REGULATION:**	Continued use of transitional objects

YOUR TOOLS	
YOUR INTERVIEW:	*Tell me about family meals with your little one. What foods does he like to eat and how is food introduction going?* *Tell me how you and the family are adjusting to having a 1-year-old in the house.* *How do you handle behaviors that you are displeased with? What behaviors does she do that just warm your heart?* *What does your nighttime or nap time routine look like now?*
YOUR OBSERVATIONS:	The adventurous explorer is now cruising with increased speed and agility and may even be standing alone or taking those first steps. His lordotic spine gives the illusion of a potbelly, while his wide-based gait and instability may appear to be a bit bowlegged. While stranger anxious and hiding behind his parents' legs, he engages with his parents by pointing at objects of interest or even those he desires and may squeak out 1–3 other words or animal sounds when enjoying a book with a caregiver.

PHYSICAL EXAM:		**COMPLETE PHYSICAL EXAM WITH A SPECIFIC FOCUS ON**	**NORMAL FINDINGS YOU MIGHT SEE AT THIS AGE**
	HEAD:	Palpate fontanelles	Anterior fontanelle open for 70%–80% of infants
	EYES:	Note red reflexes Assessment for strabismus, ocular mobility	
	MOUTH:	Inspect tonsils, palate, and erupted teeth for signs of early childhood caries (demineralization, decay)	4–8 teeth Development of geographic tongue
	CHEST:	Auscultate for murmurs, adventitious lung sounds	
	ABDOMEN:	Palpate for masses, HSM Palpate femoral pulses bilaterally	
	MSK/NEURO:	Perform Ortolani and Barlow maneuvers until toddler is walking alone or is 12 months Evaluate gait, stance, balance	Wide-based gait; unsteady balance; intoeing; bowlegged appearance
	REFLEXES:	Assess for Babinski and patellar reflexes	Faded Babinski
	GENITALIA:	Labial adhesions (♀) Circumcision vs. not, 2 descended testes (♂)	
	SKIN:	Lesions, rashes, bruising, birthmarks	Bruising consistent with falls from uncoordinated walking

YOUR TOOLS	
SCREENINGS: Screening for lead poisoning Screening for iron-deficiency anemia Tuberculosis (TB) risk assessment	*Optional based on history/risks/practice preference* Developmental screening Postpartum depression screening Oral health risk assessment (if no dental home established)
IMMUNIZATIONS: MMR #1 Hib #4 VAR #1 PCV13 #4 HepA #1 Influenza, if seasonally appropriate	

Determination, Drooling, and Da-Da (9–12 Months)
Anticipatory guidance at this stage centers on these three Ds—vitamin D, discipline, and do's & don'ts

ANTICIPATORY GUIDANCE:		
	NUTRITION:	Encourage continued breastfeeding as long as mutually desirable Change to vitamin D-fortified whole milk Continue to offer wide variety of whole foods, natural foods, but no juice or sugar-sweetened beverages
	ELIMINATION:	Diaper rash is common, so encourage use of barrier creams and seek care if rash remains present for >3 days
	SLEEP:	Sleep routine is extremely important Discuss crib safety and fall prevention from climbing out of the crib
	TRAJECTORY:	Growth expectations → Growth slows after 1st birthday Upcoming milestones → Increasing vocabulary, understanding simple commands, walking well, and stacking blocks
	SAFETY:	Discuss the difference between discipline and punishment (discipline is teaching about unwanted behavior whereas punishment is control over a bad behavior via fear). Recommend the use of redirection and time outs (1 minute per year in age) Do's & don'ts for parents: • Do provide safe spaces for exploration • Do use gates on stairs • Do keep choking hazards out of the child's reach (e.g., plastic bags, small toy parts, grapes, hot dogs, carrots, popcorn, nuts, etc.) • Don't leave the child unattended • Don't smoke around the child, including in the car • Don't use walkers, as they are a fall risk

INFANTS

12 Months

NUTRITION	
NATURAL FOODS:	• Encourage continued breastfeeding, if mutually desirable • Slowed growth now, so a decrease in appetite expected • 3 meals a day with 2–3 snacks given on a regular schedule (may skip meals and food jags are common) • Using utensils with more dexterity, but prefers finger foods • Should be adding in increasing variety of meats, poultry, beans, and fish over time • Continue to introduce wide variety of foods, including fruits, veggies with new flavors and textures
VITAMINS:	Continue vitamin D–fortified whole milk Other vitamin supplements not necessary, if eating balanced diet
IRON SOURCES:	Red meats, fish, beans Limit milk to ≤24 oz/day to prevent iron-deficiency anemia
GRAINS:	Whole-grain pasta, Cheerios, crackers are good sources
ADDED SUGAR/SALT:	Discourage added sugar, salt, sugar-sweetened beverages; limit 100% fruit juice to <4 oz/day[38] (may offer diluted with water)
TEETH:	Usually with 8 teeth; routine oral health care should be established and continue with parental assistance
DAIRY:	Should be transitioned to 16–24 oz of whole cow's milk *in a cup* unless cow's milk is contraindicated, or family prefers other form of dairy or "milk"
ELIMINATION	
OUTPUT:	Typically still in diapers, but may begin to transition to pull-ups
SLEEP	
POSITION:	Squirmy sleepers
QUANTITY:	Full night of sleep; 1–2 naps of 1–3 hours each; total: 11–14 hours May have dreams or nightmares that wake them from sleep
ROUTINE:	Pacifier has ideally been discontinued[36] Strong bedtime routine in place that includes oral health care and literacy routine
SLEEP SITE & SAFETY:	If crawling out of the crib, even on the lowest mattress setting, may need to transition to toddler bed or bed with side rails
TRACKING	
GROWTH:	Gains about 5 pounds and 4–5 inches between 12 and 24 months, so would average 2.5 pounds and 2.5 inches by 18 months[41]

FAMILY

FAMILY, INCLUDING SIBLINGS & OUTSIDE SUPPORTS:	Begin to query family about plans for additional children (recommended minimum interconception interval is 15–18 months) Ask about whether there is any noted sibling rivalry Toddler play groups; adult friends with children of the same age
ADJUSTMENT TO AGE OR STAGE:	Toddler's independence and mobility may lead to power struggles Stranger anxiety Temper tantrums, breath holding, biting, hitting
MONEY:	Continue to inquire about health and dental insurance coverage Provide information on local food banks, day care assistance programs, and other social programs if family is living below the federal poverty level
SAFETY:	Discipline philosophy/tactics Ask about consistent limits/expectations/discipline practices Is the child witnessing violence in the home, on TV, or between other adults? Ask about secondhand smoke, vaping, THC exposure, as well as revisit other substance abuse issues

LEARNING

PHYSICAL DEVELOPMENT

	15 months	*18 months*		*15 months*	*18 months*
GROSS MOTOR:	Walks well (wide gait) Stoops and recovers	Runs well Walks up steps holding hand	**FINE MOTOR:**	Stacks 2 blocks Drinks from a cup with help	Stacks 2–3 blocks Uses spoon and cup (no spills)

COMMUNICATION/LANGUAGE DEVELOPMENT

	15 months	*18 months*		
VERBAL:	3–10 meaningful words	15–20 words with 2-word phrases	**NONVERBAL:**	Brings objects to adults to show or ask for help

COGNITIVE/INTELLECTUAL DEVELOPMENT

	15 months	*18 months*		
INTELLIGENCE:	Understands simple commands	Follows simple command (no cues) Points to 1 body part	**PROBLEM-SOLVING:**	Indicates wants by pulling, pointing, or grunting

SOCIAL–EMOTIONAL DEVELOPMENT

	15 months	*18 months*		*15 months*	*18 months*
CONNECTION:	Separation anxiety continues	Kisses and feeds dolls or plush toys Explores with parents nearby	**SELF-REGULATION:**	Unpredictable behavior	Cries when toys taken away

YOUR TOOLS

YOUR INTERVIEW:	*What 3 words would you use to describe your child's personality?* *Tell me about how you are feeling about the idea of toilet training.* *How do you balance the need for keeping your child safe with allowing her to explore and try new things?* *What types of things seem to trigger temper tantrums for your child?*
YOUR OBSERVATIONS:	At 15 months, you may see a timid, fearful child with so much stranger apprehension that she plays alone and only speaks a few select words, but by 18 months, she becomes a cautious explorer who walks upstairs with confidence, "cares for" her dolls and stuffed animals, and has a vocabulary of about 18 words.

		COMPLETE PHYSICAL EXAM WITH A SPECIFIC FOCUS ON	NORMAL FINDINGS YOU MIGHT SEE AT THIS AGE
PHYSICAL EXAM:	**HEAD:**	Palpate cranial bones and for fontanelles	Anterior fontanelle still open in 40%–60% of toddlers but may be difficult to palpate
	EYES:	Note red reflexes Assess ocular mobility, strabismus, alignment	
	MOUTH:	Inspect oropharynx, teeth, and tongue	Eruption of 1st lower molar Geographic tongue
	CHEST:	Auscultate for murmurs	
	ABDOMEN:	Palpate for masses, HSM Palpate femoral pulses bilaterally	
	MSK/NEURO:	Evaluate gait, stance, balance, and strength	Wide-based gait Bowlegged appearance Stranger avoidance
	REFLEXES:	Assess patellar, Achilles, biceps, triceps, and/or brachioradialis reflexes	Disappearance of the Babinski reflex
	GENITALIA:	Labial adhesions (♀) Circumcision vs. not, 2 descended testes (♂)	
	SKIN:	Rashes, bruising, birthmarks	Café au lait spots or new nevi around 18 months

YOUR TOOLS		
SCREENINGS:	Developmental screening at 18 months Autism screening at 18 months Oral health risk assessment (if no dental home established)	*Optional based on history/risks/practice preference* Developmental screening at 15 months Iron deficiency anemia screening, if risk factors
IMMUNIZATIONS:	DTaP #4 (15 months) HepA #2 (18 months) Influenza, if seasonally appropriate	
ANTICIPATORY GUIDANCE:	**Exploration, Exuberance, and Early Childhood (15–18 Months)** In addition to safety, this stage centers on the 3 Es—elimination, exploration, and early literacy	
	NUTRITION:	Remind parents that mealtimes are when children do exploring of their food. It will become less messy once a child masters the use of utensils and that mastery comes only with continued practice. Families should provide toddlers with appropriately sized utensils for practice at meals and snack time Educate on normal nature of food jags and how best to handle them Continue iron-fortified cereals until 2 years old, if not eating other iron-rich foods regularly
	ELIMINATION:	Toilet training can begin when toddler is developmentally ready, which is signaled by interest and desire to learn, staying dry for 2-hour periods, being able to pull pants down and up, knowing the difference between wet and dry, and communicating when he needs to have a bowel movement
	SLEEP:	Transitioning to toddler bed or bed with side rails is usually a good idea from a safety perspective
	TRAJECTORY:	Reading aloud is the single most important factor in early literacy development, which correlates to increased expressive and receptive language skills, reading ability, and academic success Exploration of the world through books engages toddlers, but their ability to focus and sit is limited Upcoming milestones → Toilet training, increasing vocabulary, imitating adults in pretend play, parallel play, and improved fluency on stairs and flat surfaces
	SAFETY:	Toddlers should be given safe spaces to explore and structured outdoor play Watch toddlers closely, as fearlessness and exuberance can lead to falls and injuries Remind parents to use locks on cabinets, keep poisons out of lower cabinets, and store medications out of child's reach

NUTRITION

NATURAL FOODS:	Encourage continued breastfeeding, if mutually desirable, although most have weaned • Keep regular schedule of meals and snacks (3 meals and 2–3 snacks a day) • Continue to introduce new flavors and textures • 1 cup of fruits and 1 cup of vegetables per day[42]
VITAMINS:	Usually no supplements are needed if offering food at regular meal and snack time and the child is eating a complete diet
IRON SOURCES:	Recommended dietary allowance (RDA) is 7 mg/day; 2–3 oz/day of meat, eggs and beans*
GRAINS:	3 oz/day with 1.5 oz from whole grain sources^
ADDED SUGAR/SALT:	Limit juice to <4 oz/day Gradually begin decreasing fat intake by limiting sweets, fast-food, "snack-foods"
TEETH:	Usually with 16 teeth; routine twice daily parental brushing should continue with the addition of once daily parent-led flossing when the child has 2 teeth that are touching[43]
DAIRY:	Transition to reduced-fat milk Recommended daily intake is 2 servings/day of 1–2% or skim milk or yogurt (8 oz) or cheese (1 ½ oz natural cheese)

ELIMINATION/EXERCISE

OUTPUT:	Likely transitioned to pull-ups, but may not be fully toilet-trained during day or night
EXERCISE:	Unlimited play time in a safe environment with <1–2 hours/day of quality TV programming

SLEEP

POSITION:	Squirmy sleepers, so need to be placed in safe sleep environment; usually transitioned to a toddler bed or bed with side rails
QUANTITY:	7–8 hours/night; 1 nap of up to 3 hours in length; total: 11–14 hours May have dreams and nightmares/night terrors
ROUTINE:	Routine should be well established and include oral health care, regular bedtime, bedtime stories No TV or screens prior to bed
SLEEP SITE & SAFETY:	Bedroom safety (no blind cords within reach, cover electrical outlets, secure furniture in the room to walls, safeguard sharp furniture edges with covers, and remove items that could pose a choking hazard)

TRACKING

GROWTH:	Can expect the child to be ½ adult height and 4× birth weight

*1 oz = 1 oz of meat, poultry, or fish, ¼ cup of cooked dry beans, or 1 egg
^1 oz = 1 slice of bread, 1 cup of ready-to-eat cereal, ½ cup of cooked rice, pasta, or hot cereal

TODDLERS AND PRESCHOOLERS

FAMILY

FAMILY, INCLUDING SIBLINGS & OUTSIDE SUPPORTS:	Parental consistency around setting limits and discipline Parental time for self and partner Special time designated for family activities
	Ask about support networks (e.g., other family members, caregivers, friends, etc.) Childcare, if applicable
ADJUSTMENT TO AGE OR STAGE:	How is the family handling or reacting to temper tantrums? Balancing child's independence with safety and limit setting Toilet training success and setbacks Any newfound fears or continued stranger anxiety
MONEY:	If not asked about at the last visit, inquire about food, housing, or utility insecurity Ask about federal nutritional supplement program participation (WIC, SNAP, etc.)
SAFETY:	May be a good time to ask about firearms in the home Could ask about how safe does the family feel in their current living situation Ask about secondhand smoke, vaping, THC exposure

LEARNING

PHYSICAL DEVELOPMENT

GROSS MOTOR:	Goes up and down stairs one at a time Throws a ball overhand Jumps up	**FINE MOTOR:**	Stacks 5–6 blocks Imitates horizontal or circular strokes Can help to put clothes on

COMMUNICATION/LANGUAGE DEVELOPMENT

VERBAL:	20–50 words 2-word phrases ½ speech is understandable	**NONVERBAL:**	May revert to crying, biting, and hitting when frustrated or upset

COGNITIVE/INTELLECTUAL DEVELOPMENT

INTELLIGENCE:	Follows 2-step commands Names 1 picture in a book (cat, dog, boy)	**PROBLEM-SOLVING:**	Points to specific object when asked, "Where is…?"

SOCIAL–EMOTIONAL DEVELOPMENT

CONNECTION:	Pretend play increases Parallel play (playing alongside another toddler, but not with)	**SELF-REGULATION:**	Attachment to objects

YOUR TOOLS		
YOUR INTERVIEW:	*How many times a week do you eat family meals together?* *How is toilet training going?* *What is your child doing right now that you enjoy the most? What behaviors are most difficult?* *Tell me about the activities your child likes most.* *What changes or stresses are occurring currently for you, your child, or your family?*	
YOUR OBSERVATIONS:	The outwardly independent 2-year-old has a "me do it" attitude but can also be shy and still apprehensive of strange adults. To keep fear at bay, the child may continue to use a transitional object. When given choices, he may need time to ponder the options and a "no" answer is typically an expected answer when asking a 2-year-old if he wants to go somewhere, do something, or have someone help him.	
PHYSICAL EXAM:	**COMPLETE PHYSICAL EXAM WITH A SPECIFIC FOCUS ON**	**NORMAL FINDINGS YOU MIGHT SEE AT THIS AGE**
	VITALS: Typically move to a standing height with the use of a stadiometer; can begin calculating BMI	
	HEAD: Evaluate for trauma Palpate fontanelles	Closed anterior fontanelle (~90% are closed by 2 years of age)
	EYES: Note red reflexes Assess ocular mobility and alignment	
	MOUTH: Inspect uvula, palate, teeth, and gums	Geographic tongue
	CHEST: Auscultate for murmurs	Still's murmur
	ABDOMEN: Palpate for masses, HSM Palpate femoral pulses bilaterally	
	MSK/NEURO: Assess gait, stance, balance, and strength Observe gross and fine motor skills Note level and clarity of verbal communication	Wide-based gait Bow-legged appearance Ability to follow commands
	REFLEXES: Patellar, Achilles, biceps, triceps, and/or brachioradialis	

TODDLERS AND PRESCHOOLERS

2 Years

YOUR TOOLS		
SCREENINGS:	Autism screening Lead toxicity screening, if indicated by risk factors Iron-deficiency anemia screening, if indicated by risk factors Oral health risk assessment (if no dental home established)	*Optional based on history/risks/practice preference* Developmental screening TB risk assessment Fasting lipid panel for dyslipidemia, if (+) screen
IMMUNIZATIONS:	Influenza, if seasonally appropriate	
ANTICIPATORY GUIDANCE:	**Exploration, Exuberance, and Early Childhood (24 Months)** In addition to safety, this stage centers on these 3 Es—eating, exercise, and early childhood education (ECE)	
	NUTRITION:	Encourage continued exploration of food. Remind caregivers that it can take up to 10–15 times of exposure to a food before determining whether child "liked" or "disliked" the food Continue to encourage whole foods that are rich in iron, as well as iron-fortified foods Eliminate portion sizes distortion and encourage appropriate meal portions and frequency (2 tablespoons of each plated food group, ¼ cup or slice of grain, ½ cup or 4 oz of dairy) Avoid offering foods with choking potential (e.g., popcorn, hard candies, nuts, hot dogs, raw vegetables, and hard fruits, such as whole grapes, apples, and raisins)
	ELIMINATION:	Review signs of toilet-training readiness (see 15–18 months)
	SLEEP:	Remind parents about bedroom safety Discuss the transition to safe sleep environment
	TRAJECTORY:	Begin conversation about formal ECE programs, as many require enrollment early due to long waitlists Limit screen time to 1–2 hours and encourage 60 minutes of physical activity Upcoming milestones → Begins imaginary play, increasing communication clarity, more cooperative participation in dressing, bathing, and oral health care
	SAFETY:	Family can usually change to forward-facing car seat in the back seat, but this may vary by state Water safety and swim lessons are good to discuss at this age Discuss gun safety (ideally store guns out of the house, but if that is not an option, store guns in a locked cabinet with safety in place. Ammunition should be stored separately) Power struggles are not uncommon—offer de-escalating tips

NUTRITION

NATURAL FOODS:	Highly active, so kids continue with 3 meals a day and 2–3 snacks a day • Should keep regular schedule of meals and snacks to avoid grazing and overeating throughout the day • May become picky eaters or get stuck on a food for several days • 1 cup of vegetables and 1 cup of fruits a day
VITAMINS:	No supplements necessary if eating a complete diet
IRON SOURCES:	2–3 oz/day of meat and beans*
GRAINS:	3–4 oz/day with ½ coming from whole-grain sources^
ADDED SUGAR/SALT:	Not recommended for preschoolers, but OK to have occasional treats Limit sugar-sweetened beverages to no more than 4 oz/day (dilute)
TEETH:	Usually have all primary teeth erupted (20 teeth) by 3 years old Recommend brushing with larger, pea-sized amount of fluorinated toothpaste twice a day; continue parental flossing daily
DAIRY:	Recommended daily intake is 2 servings/day of 1% or skim milk or yogurt (8 oz) or cheese (1 ½ oz natural cheese)

ELIMINATION/EXERCISE

OUTPUT:	Typically eliminating independently, but may not be dry at night yet
EXERCISE	Unlimited active playtime with no more than 1–2 hours of quality TV/video programming per day

SLEEP

POSITION:	Continue to be somewhat squirmy sleepers, so continued use of toddler bed or guard rails for preventing falls from bed
QUANTITY:	1 nap of 1–2 hours in length; total: 10–13 hours mostly all at night
ROUTINE:	Consistent bedtime with routine May need a transitional object (e.g., a blankie or a plush toy)
SLEEP SITE & SAFETY:	Bedroom safety measures include safe sleep surfaces, attention to potential suffocation and asphyxiation hazards, securing furniture to prevent tipping/crush injuries

TRACKING

GROWTH:	Weight gains may be slower than height gains, which lead to a loss of "baby fat" and a slender appearance in the upper body Begin checking and tracking BP at 3 years old
INTERVAL HISTORY:	Any significant illnesses, changes in medical or family history should be noted

*1 oz = 1 oz of meat, poultry, or fish, ¼ cup of cooked dry beans, or 1 egg
^1 oz = 1 slice of bread, 1 cup of ready-to-eat cereal, ½ cup of cooked rice, pasta, or hot cereal

TODDLERS AND PRESCHOOLERS

FAMILY

FAMILY, INCLUDING SIBLINGS & OUTSIDE SUPPORTS:	How do working parents make time for each other and for dedicated family activities? Balancing roles of working and parenting Play with siblings (sharing/turn-taking); sibling rivalry Preschool educators; toddler play groups; scheduled activities (e.g., ballet lessons or karate classes)
ADJUSTMENT TO AGE OR STAGE:	Transition to preschool, ECE, or Head Start Negotiating with parents and power struggles Activity and energy level of preschooler Attention span of a preschooler
MONEY:	Financial, food, housing, or utility insecurity Discuss continued use of WIC and/or SNAP benefits (if applicable) Provide information on day care assistance and high-quality preschool options (e.g., Head Start)
SAFETY:	Could review living situation to assess for potential safety hazards (e.g., apartment building with third floor windows, rural area with potential for farm injury, etc.) Ask about secondhand smoke, vaping, THC exposure Encourage a smoke-free environment and offer resources for cessation

LEARNING

PHYSICAL DEVELOPMENT

GROSS MOTOR:	Throws a ball overhand Balances on one foot for 1 second Pedals a tricycle	**FINE MOTOR:**	Draws a person with 2 body parts Thumb wiggle Towers 6–7 blocks

COMMUNICATION/LANGUAGE DEVELOPMENT

VERBAL:	Conversations with pronouns, plurals 2–3 sentences per idea Speech is 75% understandable

COGNITIVE/INTELLECTUAL DEVELOPMENT

INTELLIGENCE:	Names 4 pictures in a book Knows 1 color	**PROBLEM-SOLVING:**	Prepares cereal Names use of cup, ball, spoon, and crayon

SOCIAL–EMOTIONAL DEVELOPMENT

CONNECTION:	Interactive play Shows affection for friends/family	**SELF-REGULATION:**	Increasingly better at taking turns

YOUR TOOLS

YOUR INTERVIEW:	*How do you feel about this age/stage for your child?* *Tell me about how you set limits or provide choices for your child. What do you do if your child is uncooperative or pushing boundaries?* Interviewing the child becomes an option starting at 3 to 4 years old, so asking about favorite activities, books, toys, and foods is most appropriate as means of assessing the child's development, eating habits, early literacy exposures, and interests.
YOUR OBSERVATIONS:	Chatter bugs with newly acquired language skills work to negotiate with you throughout the visit. These language abilities lead to new play skills that include imaginative and interactive play. Drawings of friends may be primitive with a large head and one other body part (usually something circular, like an oval body or circular eyes). Favorite outdoor activities might include tricycle riding, tossing a ball, or practicing balancing moves.

PHYSICAL EXAM:	COMPLETE PHYSICAL EXAM WITH A SPECIFIC FOCUS ON		NORMAL FINDINGS YOU MIGHT SEE AT THIS AGE
	VITALS:	Calculating BMI Begin measuring BP (at 3 years old)	BMI >5th percentile and <85th percentile BP <90th percentile when calculated using a BP percentile calculator, such as www.mdcalc.com
	EYES:	Perform fundoscopic exam for visualization of optic nerve and vessels	Visual acuity at 20/50 or better (if child cooperative and developmentally appropriate)
	NECK:	Assess for lymphadenopathy Palpate thyroid	Shotty lymph nodes not unusual
	MOUTH:	Inspect uvula, tonsils, palate, teeth, and gums	Full set of 20 primary teeth Tonsillar hypertrophy without evidence of infection Geographic tongue
	CHEST:	Auscultate for murmurs	Still's murmur or venous hum
	ABDOMEN:	Palpate for masses, HSM Palpate femoral pulses bilaterally	
	MSK/NEURO:	Assess gait, stance, balance, and strength Observe parent–child interaction, communication skills, and speech clarity	Knock-knee appearance begins around 3 years Intoeing gait in 10% of childen[44] Lumbar lordosis
	REFLEXES:	Patellar, Achilles, biceps, triceps, and/or brachioradialis	
	SKIN:	Lesions, rashes, bruising, birthmarks	Regression of cutaneous hemangiomas

YOUR TOOLS		
Screenings:	Developmental screening at 2 ½ years (30 months) Vision screening, if child is able to cooperate, with tumbling E or LEA symbols at 3 years Oral health risk assessment (if no dental home established)	*Optional based on history/risks/practice preference* Developmental screening (3 years)
Immunizations:	Typically none, but catch-up vaccines and influenza, if seasonally appropriate	
Anticipatory Guidance:	**Funny, Fickle, and Friendly (3 Years Old)** Much of the anticipatory guidance at this stage centers on these 3 Fs—foods, freedom, and firmness	
	Nutrition:	Discuss food jags as a normal developmental stage related to feeding Review portion sizes (1 tbsp for each year of age) and recommendations for feeding on a schedule with food offered every 2–4 hours Advise families on using the My Little Eater FFPP model for meal planning. This includes having a source of fiber, healthy fat, protein, and produce at every meal[45] Eliminate mealtime fights by having parents decide what variety of healthy foods to offer at a meal and allowing the child to decide how much, if any, to eat
	Elimination & Exercise:	When preschooler doesn't stop activity to attend to bowel/bladder function, it's not unusual to have occasional daytime accidents Recommend unlimited unstructured activity with screen time limited to 1–2 hours
	Sleep:	Routine and limit setting around sleep continue to be important Remind parents that children may wake due to dreams, nightmares, and night terrors
	Trajectory:	Encourage continued reading aloud and provide community resources (e.g., library) for book acquisition Discuss preparation/readiness for preschool or ECE Upcoming milestones → Fantasy play with the ability to predict what may happen next in a story, hoping on a single foot, copying a cross, increasing speech fluency and clarity
	Safety:	Discuss struggle to balance the freedom a 3-year-old needs to explore with the limits that he needs to keep him safe, organized, and functional Remind parents that children demonstrate more desirable behaviors when given firm limits with the freedom to make choices within those limits, such as which shoes to wear out of two choices

NUTRITION

NATURAL FOODS:	1 ½ cups of vegetables and 1–1 ½ cups of fruit daily[42]
VITAMINS:	No vitamin or mineral supplementation needed if eating a balanced, complete diet with vitamin D–fortified dairy products
IRON SOURCES:	3–4 oz/day of meat and beans*[46] Limit cow's milk to ≤24 oz/day
GRAINS:	4–5 oz/day with ½ coming from whole grain sources^
ADDED SUGAR/SALT:	Limit sugar-sweetened beverages to no more than 4 oz/day (dilute)
TEETH:	Twice-daily brushing with pea-sized fluorinated toothpaste followed by parental flossing
DAIRY:	Recommended daily intake is 2 ½ servings/day of reduced fat or skim milk or yogurt (8 oz) or cheese (1 ½ oz natural cheese)

ELIMINATION/EXERCISE

OUTPUT:	Typically eliminating independently with daytime bowel and bladder control; daytime (when distracted) accidents and bedwetting are not uncommon and positive reinforcement principles should be used by the family
EXERCISE:	Should be supported to have unlimited active playtime with limited media time (1–2 hours of quality programming/day) Weekly family physical activity should be encouraged[8]

SLEEP

POSITION:	Less important at this age
QUANTITY:	Naps become less frequent; total: 10–13 hours Magical thinking in this age can bring about fear of the dark or monsters under the bed Fears can have kids waking due to nightmares (up to 50% of kids in this age have nightmares), but the less common night terrors (~30% of kids at this age) are not related to psychological issues[47] Kids with history consistent with night terrors have a higher incidence of familial association with other sleep-related disorders such as obstructive sleep apnea, restless leg syndrome, and nocturnal asthma, so involving a sleep specialist may be prudent[47]
ROUTINE:	Routine with a consistent bedtime continues to be important with emphasis on reinforcing healthy sleep hygiene
SLEEP SITE & SAFETY:	Toddler bed or bed with side rails and bedroom safety unchanged from previous recommendations

TRACKING

GROWTH:	Gains slow to an average of 4.5 pounds per year in weight and 3 inches in height
INTERVAL HISTORY:	Any significant illnesses, changes in medical or family history should be noted

*1 oz = 1 oz of meat, poultry, or fish, ¼ cup of cooked dry beans, or 1 egg
^1 oz = 1 slice of bread, 1 cup of ready-to-eat cereal, ½ cup of cooked rice, pasta, or hot cereal

FAMILY

FAMILY, INCLUDING SIBLINGS & OUTSIDE SUPPORTS:	Ask about family planning Work-life-parenting balance ECE facilities/educators; role of neighbors, extended family
ADJUSTMENT TO AGE OR STAGE:	Child's ability to get along with other children Pushing limits Energy level and need for physical activities
MONEY:	Any financial, housing, food, or utility insecurity? Continue to encourage the use of WIC until child is 5 years old, if needed and qualify
SAFETY:	Inquire about violence exposures for caregiver(s) or children Ask about exposure to secondhand smoke, vaping, THC exposure Encourage smoke-free environment and offer resources for smoking cessation

LEARNING

PHYSICAL DEVELOPMENT

GROSS MOTOR:	Hops Pedals a bike with training wheels Dresses and undresses without assistance	**FINE MOTOR:**	Mature pencil grasp Copies a cross or circle Draws a person with 2–4 body parts

COMMUNICATION/LANGUAGE DEVELOPMENT

VERBAL:	Tells a story Talkative with animated conversations Speech is 100% understandable

COGNITIVE/INTELLECTUAL DEVELOPMENT

INTELLIGENCE:	Defines 5 words and counts up to 5 Knows 4 colors	**PROBLEM-SOLVING:**	Plays card and board games Knows what to do if cold, hungry, or tired

SOCIAL–EMOTIONAL DEVELOPMENT

CONNECTION:	Enjoys make-believe play (magical thinking) Insatiable curiosity (asks why, when, where, how questions) Collaborative play and developing friendships	**SELF-REGULATION:**	Identifies emotions in themself

YOUR TOOLS

YOUR INTERVIEW:	*Tell me how preschool is going. What changes have you noticed since she started attending?* *Tell me about your child's role in family meal times and bedtime/nap time activities.* Questions you could ask the child: Ask the child about gender, age, friends, favorite activity, favorite book/movie/super hero. Ask about favorite part/activity at preschool and favorite story heard recently.
YOUR OBSERVATIONS:	Preschoolers with a widened vocabulary, imaginative play, newly developing friendships (maybe even imaginary friends), and storytelling abilities make the 4-year-old visit fun and fantasy filled. You may be able to convince the 4-year-old that only fruits and veggies will give them the ability to climb to the top of the big slide or that milk gives them super powers. Their increasing autonomy has these kids removing their princess dresses or super hero costumes with minimal parental help and separating from their caregiver for weighing, measuring, and vision screening with ease.

PHYSICAL EXAM:	COMPLETE PHYSICAL EXAM WITH A SPECIFIC FOCUS ON		NORMAL FINDINGS YOU MIGHT SEE AT THIS AGE
	VITALS:	BMI BP percentile	BMI >5th percentile and <85th percentile BP percentile <90th percentile (www.mdcalc.com)
	HEAD:	Evaluate for trauma	
	EYES:	Assess visual acuity	20/40 or better on Snellen visual acuity measures
	EARS:	Assess gross hearing Appreciate TM mobility and appearance	
	NOSE:	Inspect septum, mucosa, and turbinates	
	MOUTH:	Inspect teeth and gums	Enlarged tonsillar pillars; geographic tongue
	CHEST:	Auscultate for murmurs, palpate femoral pulses	
	ABDOMEN:	Palpate for masses, HSM	Still's and venous hum murmurs
	MSK/NEURO:	Assess gait, stance, balance, and strength Observe fine motor skills with paper and crayons Observe communication, speech, cognition	Mature pencil grasp for some activities with reverting to immature grasp for other tasks Upwards of 30% of kids have an intoeing gait[44]
	REFLEXES:	Patellar, Achilles, biceps, triceps, and/or brachioradialis	Fear, uncooperativeness with reflex exam Exaggerated or diminished reflexes may be present due to cooperation

YOUR TOOLS

SCREENINGS:	Auditory screening Oral health risk assessment (if no dental home established) Vision screening	*Optional based on history/risks/practice preference* Developmental screening
IMMUNIZATIONS:	IPV#4 DTaP #5 MMR #2	VAR #2 Influenza, if seasonally appropriate

Gregarious, Goofy, and Getting Ready (4 Years Old)
The anticipatory guidance for 4-year-old WCCs may focus on gun safety, grown-ups, and getting ready for school

ANTICIPATORY GUIDANCE:		
	NUTRITION:	Food portions for a 4-year-old are approximately a ½ of a whole piece of fruit or ½ cup, ½ cup of vegetable, 1 oz of protein and 1 oz of grain (preferably whole grains) for each meal and snack. All but one snack can be accompanied by 4 oz of dairy[42] Using a sensible feeding system found on a website like mylittleeater.com, balanced meals should contain a serving size of fiber, fat, protein, and produce, while snacks may contain any three out of the four macronutrients[45]
	ELIMINATION & EXERCISE:	Most children are daytime toilet trained by 4 years old, with 85% of kids reaching nighttime dryness by 5 years old
	SLEEP:	Routine and limit setting around sleep should continue Warn parents that children may wake due to dreams, nightmares, and night terrors
	TRAJECTORY:	Following routines, playing games that include identifying letters and sounds, reading with children, and providing age-appropriate chores will help develop skills to attend school Upcoming milestones → Counting to 10, tells a simple story with correct tenses and pronouns, prints letters and numbers, hopping and skipping
	SAFETY:	Cover gun safety, including safe storage (out of the house or locked with the safety in place and ammunition in separate storage area) Discuss responding to grown-up strangers and "good touch/bad touch" (private areas are those covered by a bathing suit, no adults should ask kids to help with their private parts, etc.)

NUTRITION

NATURAL FOODS:	3 meals a day with 1–2 snacks a day 1 ½ cups[+] of vegetables and fruits daily
VITAMINS:	Supplemental vitamins are not usually necessary if child has no underlying medical issues and eats a complete, balanced diet
IRON SOURCES:	3–4 oz/day of meat and beans*
GRAINS:	4–5 oz/day with ½ coming from whole-grain sources^
ADDED SUGAR/SALT:	Limit sugar-sweetened beverages to no more than 4 oz/day
TEETH:	Usually begin to lose primary teeth at 5 to 6 years old in the same order that they erupted Child may have improved brushing technique and may start brushing once to twice a day independently, but parent-assisted flossing should continue once daily
DAIRY:	Recommended daily intake is 2–2 ½ servings/day of 1% or skim milk or yogurt (8 oz) or cheese (1 ½ oz natural cheese)

ELIMINATION/EXERCISE

OUTPUT:	Nocturnal enuresis resolved in 85% of children, but 15% are still wetting the bed at night at 5 years old
EXERCISE:	60 minutes of exercise daily Bike safety and helmets should be used regularly

SLEEP

POSITION:	Typically have moved to a regular bed
QUANTITY:	10–12 hours/night; 0–1 nap; total: 10–13 hours
ROUTINE:	Wake up around 6–8 am; typical bedtime is 7–8 pm Routines are still important, but have likely changed with start of school
SLEEP HYGIENE:	Should not be using electronics within an hour of bedtime, as blue light from devices affects the production of melatonin[48] A warm bath 1–2 hours prior to sleep decreases the time to sleep and increases sleep depth and increases non-REM consolidation, which is when the body repairs and regenerates tissues, builds bone and muscle, and improves immune system[49]

TRACKING

GROWTH:	Height velocities decelerate to ~6 cm/year (2.5 inches) and track within a growth channel without crossing percentile lines[50] Weight gains can vary between 4–7 pounds per year[51] but typically average about 5 pounds a year
INTERVAL HISTORY:	Any significant illnesses, changes in medical or family history should be noted

[+]½ cup = 1 serving
*1 oz = 1 oz of meat, poultry, or fish, ¼ cup of cooked dry beans, or 1 egg
^1 oz = 1 slice of bread, 1 cup of ready-to-eat cereal, ½ cup of cooked rice, pasta, or hot cereal

SCHOOL-AGE CHILDREN

FAMILY

Family, Including Siblings & Outside Supports:	Ask about family expectations around school performance, household participation, and chores Starting kindergarten, so working with school as a support Increased interest in spending time with friends rather than family After-school care arrangements
Adjustment to Age or Stage:	Transition to kindergarten; socially and academically Any sense of loss or anxiety for parents around this transition Adhering to a schedule and new routines Testing previously established rules and anger and impulse control difficulties
Money:	Continue to ask about financial insecurity (Trouble making ends meet? Trouble paying for heat, electricity, phone?) WIC benefits end at age of 5, but depending on income, child may qualify for free or reduced breakfast and lunch programs
Safety:	Ask about feeling safe in the house, at school, and in the neighborhood Begin asking the child about their smoke exposures and knowledge about health dangers associated with tobacco use Continue to encourage a smoke-free environment and resources for parents/caregivers interested in cessation

LEARNING

Physical Development

Gross Motor:	Hops and skips Climbs trees Tests physical ability	**Fine Motor:**	Draws a person with 6+ body parts Prints some letters and numbers Copies a square at 5 and a triangle at 6

Communication/Language Development

Verbal:	Good articulation and accelerated expressive language Storytelling using appropriate tenses and pronouns

Cognitive/Intellectual Development

Intelligence:	Can count to 10+ Begins to understand number concepts Magical thinking mixed with concrete thinking	**Problem-Solving:**	Begins to sequence and organize Basic adding and subtracting

Social–Emotional Development

Connection:	Explores gender identity Cooperative (sharing) play Expresses positive and negative feelings for family members	**Self-Regulation:**	Slowly improving impulse control Understands need for rules Obeys rules

YOUR TOOLS

YOUR INTERVIEW:	*What has been the most surprising thing you've noticed about your child since your child started school?* *How do you think the transition to school is going?* *Does her teacher have any concerns about her performance/progress in school? How was the last parent–teacher conference?* *Questions you could ask the child: What is your favorite story to read right now? What do you and your friends like to do when together? What part of school do you like the most? What do you like the least? What games do you play at recess and who do you play with? What is the first thing you do when you get on your bike (or into the car)?*
YOUR OBSERVATIONS:	The rule follower is much better at paying attention, adhering to instructions and attending to others. However, their egocentric thinking and imagination still dominates. Wanting to show off their physical prowess, they will be happy to show you how they can balance on a single foot, hop down the hall, or flex their muscles. They are also intent on showing you their new-found academic skills. Counting to 10, printing their name and maybe even drawing you a picture of their family are easy in-office observations to gauge school readiness or progress.

PHYSICAL EXAM:	COMPLETE PHYSICAL EXAM WITH A SPECIFIC FOCUS ON		NORMAL FINDINGS YOU MIGHT SEE AT THIS AGE
	VITALS:	BMI BP percentile	BMI >5th percentile and <85th percentile BP percentile <90th percentile (www.mdcalc.com)
	HEAD:	Evaluate for trauma	
	EYES:	Visual acuity EOM and fundoscopic exam	20/30 or better
	EARS:	Inspect TMs	
	MOUTH	Inspect tonsils, teeth, and gums	Tonsillar enlargement
	CHEST:	Auscultate for adventitious sounds, murmurs, palpate femoral pulses	Innocent flow murmurs
	ABDOMEN:	Palpate for masses, HSM	
	MSK/NEURO:	Assess gait, stance, balance, and strength	
	REFLEXES:	Patellar, Achilles, biceps, triceps, and/or brachioradialis	

SCHOOL-AGE CHILDREN

YOUR TOOLS		
SCREENINGS:	Auditory screening Oral health risk assessment (if no dental home established) Vision screening Psychosocial/behavioral assessment	*Optional based on history/risks/practice preference* Developmental screening
IMMUNIZATIONS:	Typically none, but catch-up vaccines and influenza, if seasonally appropriate	
ANTICIPATORY GUIDANCE:	**Honing, Habits, and Heading off to School (5–6 Years Old)** The anticipatory guidance for this stage centers on homework, helmets, and healthy habits	
	NUTRITION:	Healthy habits to reinforce include incorporating a fruit or vegetable into each of the 3 meals and as 1–2 snacks during the day, eating a healthy breakfast, and avoiding sugar-sweetened beverages and instead offering reduced-fat milk with 2 meals a day
	EXERCISE:	Encourage 60 minutes per day of moderate to vigorous physical activity (MVPA) with <2 hour of leisure screen time Discuss development of self-efficacy through team sports and appropriate parental support
	SLEEP:	Nighttime enuresis, if present, usually improves at rate of 5% each year, so of the 15% of kids with nocturnal enuresis at 5 years old, 5% will become dry within the next year Routine with regular bedtime and awakening times helps improve school performance
	TRAJECTORY:	Create routines around homework to reinforce concepts being taught in school (reading nightly even if it isn't assigned, helping with homework, but not doing it for them, creating a space and a time in the routine to do the homework, etc.) Upcoming milestones → Increasing independence, coordination, vocabulary, and memory; thinking becomes concrete, reversible, and able to consider 2 or more aspects of a problem
	SAFETY:	Remind patients that the use of a helmet is recommended whenever on wheels (bike, scooter, skateboard, and roller skates) Discuss the appropriateness of moving to a booster seat with a lap belt Supervise children crossing the street until at least 8–9 years old, as ability to judge distance, speed, and location of sounds not yet fully developed in this school-aged brain

5 & 6 Years

NUTRITION

NATURAL FOODS:	Nutritional requirements will vary by age, diet type, and activity level, but on average the most sedentary children need: 1 ½ cups[+] of vegetables and 1–1 ½ cups[+] fruit every day
VITAMINS:	Supplemental vitamins are not usually necessary if child is healthy and eats a complete, balanced diet
IRON SOURCES:	3–4 oz/day of meat and beans*
GRAINS:	4–5 oz/day with ½ coming from whole grain sources^
ADDED SUGAR/SALT:	Limit sugar-sweetened beverages to no more than 4 oz/day (dilute)
TEETH:	By 8 years old, the top and bottom 4 primary incisors replaced by permanent teeth Continue oral health care routine with twice-daily brushing and daily flossing
DAIRY:	Recommended daily intake is 2 ½ servings/day of 1% or skim milk or yogurt (8 oz) or cheese (1 ½ oz natural cheese)

EXERCISE

CARDIOVASCULAR:	Recommended that children participate in 60 minutes of MVPA daily; however, a decline in MVPA begins at ~7 years of age[52] A combination of strength and skill-based activities should be encouraged using developmentally appropriate exercises, like games with animal-like movements (e.g., bear crawl, crocodile planks, flamingo stance, etc.)
STRENGTHENING:	Physical education classes and sporting activities increasingly include resistance (strength) training to increase muscle strength and reduce overuse injuries[53]

SLEEP

POSITION:	In a regular bed
QUANTITY:	10–12 hours/night; no naps; total: 9–12 hours
ROUTINE:	Wake up around 6–7 am and typical bedtime is 8–9 pm Routines, especially around waking time, important for school
SLEEP HYGIENE:	Minimize blue light and electronic use at least 1 hour prior to bedtime; no TV in bedroom

TRACKING

GROWTH:	Height velocities continue steadily at 2.5 inches per year Weight gains can vary between 4 and 7 pounds/year,[51] but typically average about 5 pounds a year
INTERVAL HISTORY:	Any significant illnesses, changes in medical or family history should be noted

[+] ½ cup = 1 serving
* 1 oz = 1 oz of meat, poultry, or fish, ¼ cup of cooked dry beans, or 1 egg
^ 1 oz = 1 slice of bread, 1 cup of ready-to-eat cereal, ½ cup of cooked rice, pasta, or hot cereal

SCHOOL-AGE CHILDREN

FAMILY		
FAMILY, INCLUDING SIBLINGS & OUTSIDE SUPPORTS:	Family's perspective on expecting more involved chores that require more time, concentration, and attention to detail Family time with special activities May be more physically aggressive with siblings Parents of child's friends After-school care Teacher/school support	
ADJUSTMENT TO AGE OR STAGE:	Adhering to a schedule with new routines Increasing school demands Increased time with friends rather than with family	
MONEY:	Increasing importance to children, as desired items are more costly Money sometimes equated to social status and peer acceptance	
SAFETY:	Bullying and/or physical fights at school Neighborhood safety Firearms in the home Begin asking the child about their smoke and tobacco exposures, knowledge about health dangers associated with tobacco use Continue to encourage a smoke-free environment and resources for parents/caregivers interested in cessation	
LEARNING		

PHYSICAL DEVELOPMENT

GROSS MOTOR:	Improved eye-hand coordination[54] Adult levels of balance and postural control[55]	

COMMUNICATION/LANGUAGE DEVELOPMENT

VERBAL:	Increased vocabulary Can tell a coherent narrative with beginning, middle, and end	

COGNITIVE/INTELLECTUAL DEVELOPMENT

INTELLIGENCE:	Two-directional (reversible) thinking Improved memory	**PROBLEM-SOLVING:** Ability to consider 2 or more aspects of a problem Improved perspective taking

SOCIAL–EMOTIONAL DEVELOPMENT

CONNECTION:	Fantasy play becomes internalized Wider net of same gender friends	**SELF-REGULATION:** Increased coping skills Increasing control over feelings

YOUR TOOLS

YOUR INTERVIEW:	*Do you have any concerns about your child's progress in school?* *What has been your family's approach to dividing up household chores/responsibilities?* *In what ways do you allow your child to contribute to family decisions, like the movie to watch or the type of food to eat?* *When she breaks a rule, what consequences do you enforce?* *Questions you could ask the child: Do you have a best friend? How are you doing in school this year? How do you feel about that performance? What is your favorite vegetable? How often do you eat it? What is the rule in your house about watching TV or playing video games?*
YOUR OBSERVATIONS:	At this age, children are beginning to see that there is a whole world around them and that they are not necessarily at the center of that world. They also realize that this surrounding world has socially appropriate rules that can vary by the situation. They may demonstrate this by climbing up and down off the exam table until you come into the room, at which time they may stop this behavior and conform to the norm of "sitting still and talking with the provider." You may be escorted into the room by a child who holds the door open for you and he may hand you the wall-mounted otoscope, all while telling you all about the rules of the action-figure wars or the latest trading card games that are played at recess. The logical and curious cognitive development may drive her to want to know more about how the equipment works and why we use it. They are beginning to think with more reason and analysis, so you may find them telling you what you are going to do next in your exam and why.

PHYSICAL EXAM:		**COMPLETE PHYSICAL EXAM WITH A SPECIFIC FOCUS ON**	**NORMAL FINDINGS YOU MIGHT SEE AT THIS AGE**
	VITALS:	BMI BP percentile	BMI >5th percentile and <85th percentile BP percentile <90th percentile (www.mdcalc.com)
	GENERAL:	Activity level, maturity, and interaction with parents/adults	Shy children may appear less mature
	EYES:	Assess visual fields, visual acuity, EOMs	20/30 or better
	MOUTH:	Inspect tonsils, teeth, and gums	Early evidence of malocclusions may be obvious
	CHEST:	Assess for breast development and Tanner stage	Tanner II breast development as early as 8
	MSK/NEURO:	Observe LE joint function (hip, knee, and ankle)	5%–9% of school-aged kids will have adducted (intoeing) gait[44]
	GENITALIA:	SMR	No pubic hair development
	SKIN:	Evidence of early pubertal development	Axillary hair, comedomal acne, and increased oil on the face and upper back

SCHOOL-AGE CHILDREN

YOUR TOOLS		
SCREENINGS:	Auditory screening (8 years old) Psychosocial/behavioral assessment Vision screening (8 years old)	*Optional based on history/risks/practice preference* Developmental screening
IMMUNIZATIONS:	Annual flu immunization and catch-up immunizations as needed	

ANTICIPATORY GUIDANCE:

Independent, Inventive, and Inquisitive (7–8 Years Old)
The anticipatory guidance for this age centers on the 3 Is—internet, importance/self-esteem, and issues at school

NUTRITION:	Recommend 3 meals and 1–2 nutrient-dense snacks per day Encourage families to eat a serving of veggies or fruit at every meal and with each snack Milk intake begins to drop off, so may need to get inventive in terms of calcium intake (fortified foods, cheese, and yogurt)
EXERCISE:	Encourage at least 1 hour daily of age-appropriate play/activity that is a combination of cardiovascular and strength training Discuss participation in organized sports with appropriate parental expectations
SLEEP:	Review importance of regular bedtime and waking times Bedtime routine should not involve electronics or TV Emphasize the importance of good quality sleep on restoration, growth, and brain function
TRAJECTORY:	Identify concerns about school performance and/or praise school successes Remind parents that praising children for responsible behavior, allowing them to make age-appropriate decisions, and giving them chores will help children gain competence and see their importance to the family and the community Upcoming milestones → Improved executive functioning and problem-solving, pubertal development may begin for girls, begins to understand nuances of language
SAFETY:	Discuss bullying Provide tips on how to help the child feel important and promote a strong self-esteem Review internet safety, including supervising kids whenever they are online, allowing only age-appropriate game choices, limiting screen time, and employing internet filters Remind kids that "browsing the internet" can be potentially harmful and is not a good use of time Discuss whether child qualifies to move out of booster seat (usually 8 years old, 57", and 80 pounds)

NUTRITION

NATURAL FOODS:	Usually eating 3 meals with 1 snack Caloric intake varies by activity level, but on average require 1,600–1,800 calories a day 2–2 ½ cups+ of vegetables and 1 ½ cups+ of fruit
VITAMINS:	May need to encourage some calcium- or iron-fortified foods if meat and dairy intake is less than daily recommended intake
IRON SOURCES:	5 oz/day of meat, eggs, or beans*
GRAINS:	4–5 oz/day with ½ coming from whole-grain sources^
ADDED SUGAR/SALT:	Limit sugar-sweetened beverages, snack foods, pre-packaged lunch kits, and sugared cereals Fast-food or restaurant eating should be limited to 1×/week or less
TEETH:	Usually a 1–2 year break in permanent tooth eruption at 9 and 10 years old Continue oral health care routine with twice-daily brushing and once-daily flossing, which may begin to transition to child
DAIRY:	Recommended daily intake is 3 servings/day of reduced-fat milk or yogurt (8 oz) or cheese (1 ½ oz natural cheese)

EXERCISE

CARDIOVASCULAR:	Recommended that children participate in 60 minutes of MVPA daily Team or individual sports highly recommended for physical activity and socialization aspects
STRENGTHENING:	Increasing balance and coordination may make body weight and resistance band exercise more feasible than at a younger age[53]

SLEEP

POSITION:	Typically have moved to a regular bed
QUANTITY:	10–12 hours/night; no naps; total: 10–12 hours
ROUTINE:	Increasing independence with nighttime activities and routine Routines during the summer may be altered with no scheduled school, but highly recommend child keeps some regularity
SLEEP HYGIENE:	Child may begin bathing on a daily basis (with the onset of early pubertal changes), so bathing 1 hour prior to bedtime can help with getting to sleep sooner and staying asleep longer Kids with insomnia should not use sleep aides unless they have failed behavioral interventions. Melatonin can be used at the lowest effective dose for short-term resets of the circadian rhythm[48]

TRACKING

GROWTH:	Girls' height growth spurt begins between 9 and 10 years old
INTERVAL HISTORY:	Any interval illnesses or changes in the medical or family history should be captured

+½ cup = 1 serving
*1 oz = 1 oz of meat, poultry, or fish, ¼ cup of cooked dry beans, or 1 egg
^1 oz = 1 slice of bread, 1 cup of ready-to-eat cereal, ½ cup of cooked rice, pasta, or hot cereal

SCHOOL-AGE CHILDREN

9 & 10 Years

FAMILY

Family, Including Siblings & Outside Supports:	Family time with special activities Family functioning (strongest risk factor and strongest protective factor for behavior and learning problems) Household responsibilities with increasing complexity and that require more time, concentration, and/or attention to detail After-school activities; summer camps/summer programs Teachers or coaches
Adjustment to Age or Stage:	Increasing school demands Increasing interest and time with friends rather than family Adhering to schedule/routines
Money:	Discussing food insecurity, financial stresses, and employment of the parents Backpack programs, food pantries, SNAP benefits can be useful resources for families struggling with food insecurity
Safety:	School safety Firearm safety At 10, begin asking about personal tobacco use (cigarettes, e-cigs/vaping, chewing) and actively discuss techniques to overcome peer pressures, as well as reminding the patient of the health benefits of not using tobacco (usually best received when put in the context of a limitation on something that the child likes/wants to do, such as *"Smoking damages your lungs and you have said you want to continue swimming. How do you think that smoking might impact your lungs while swimming?"*)

LEARNING

Physical Development

Gross Motor:	Improved strength, flexibility, and physical skill

Communication/Language Development

Verbal:	Understands metaphors, similes, and figures of speech Enjoys word play and jokes

Cognitive/Intellectual Development

Intelligence:	Improved executive processing Categorizes, memorizes, and recalls more efficiently	**Problem-Solving:**	Tries new approaches to problem-solving more readily

Social–Emotional Development

Connection:	Ritualized play with friends (e.g., trading card games, team sports, recess games) Hero or role model has become a real person	**Self-Regulation:**	More adept at appraising a situation and using coping skills

YOUR TOOLS

YOUR INTERVIEW:	*Do you have any concerns about your child's progress in school?* *Have any of the child's teachers mentioned concerns about her learning, attention, concentration, or being overly active?* Questions you could ask the child: *How are you doing in school this year? What is easy about school? What do you find most difficult? What is one thing outside of school that you think you are good at? How would your friends describe you, if they only had 3–4 words? What chores do you do to help around the house?*
YOUR OBSERVATIONS:	This child is more poised and astutely aware of his surroundings and the expectations related to behavior in those surroundings. He is becoming more aware of how others see him and may use this as a comparison point when talking about how he stacks up to his peer group (e.g., "I'm in the advanced math class, but most of my friends are in the regular math class."). He may bring one of his collections or hobbies to the appointment, yet has self-control, puts the collection away when it is time for the exam. When asked about what he wants to be when he grows up, a child at this age may be able to use a metaphor, a figure of speech, or some advanced narrative to indicate that he wants to be in the same role as his real-life role model (e.g., "I'm gonna be like Michael Jordan when I grow up and sink 3s for a living.").

		COMPLETE PHYSICAL EXAM WITH A SPECIFIC FOCUS ON	NORMAL FINDINGS YOU MIGHT SEE AT THIS AGE
PHYSICAL EXAM:	**VITALS:**	BMI BP percentile	BMI stable and tracking; <85th percentile BP percentile <90th percentile (www.mdcalc.com)
	EARS:	Evaluate internal and external structures Assess hearing	Multiple ear piercings
	MOUTH:	Inspect uvula, palate teeth, and gums	No new tooth eruption
	CHEST:	Auscultate for murmurs, SMR	Tanner II–III breasts
	MSK/NEURO:	Assess gait, stance, balance, and strength Evaluate for scoliosis starting at 10 for ♀	
	REFLEXES:	Patellar, Achilles, biceps, triceps, brachioradialis	
	GENITALIA:	SMR/Tanner staging	Tanner II pubic hair development in females, but Tanner I staging for males
	SKIN:	Signs of self-inflicted trauma, lesions, piercings	Comedomal and inflammatory acne
	PSYCH:	Attention, activity level, affect, developmentally appropriate social and cognitive gains	Inattention if asked to focus for long periods of time

YOUR TOOLS

SCREENINGS:	Auditory screening (10 years old) Dyslipidemia screening (once between 9 and 11 years old) Psychosocial/behavioral assessment (depending on tool, youth may begin to self-report at age 10)	*Optional based on history/risks/practice preference* Vision screening (10 years old)
IMMUNIZATIONS:	Tdap can be given at 10 years old, but it is often deferred/held until 11-year-old WCC and administered with other vaccines Influenza, if seasonally appropriate	

ANTICIPATORY GUIDANCE:		**Independent, Inventive, and Inquisitive (9–10 Years Old)** The anticipatory guidance for this age centers on the 3 Is—internet, independence, and issues at school
	NUTRITION:	Eating breakfast everyday helps to start the day off by putting gas in the tank for your body and brain Water or white milk are the healthiest drink choices, as even juice can have as much sugar as candy bars Children can help plan and prepare parts of the family meals Encourage families to have fresh fruit and veggies on hand for lunches and after school snacks and discuss healthy snack options as kids are asked to make more of their own food choices at home and at school
	EXERCISE:	60 minutes of MVPA daily with 3 days of the week including muscle strengthening and bone strengthening exercises (resistance exercises with body weight or resistance bands, climbing on playground equipment, running, jumping rope, yoga would be appropriate for this age)[56]
	SLEEP:	Sleep routines should be reinforced, especially with increasing independence and more self-responsibility over nighttime routines No electronic devices prior to sleep and avoid violent video games to decrease sleep issues
	TRAJECTORY:	Educate on pubertal changes, hygiene, delaying sexual behavior, and encouraging questions/open forum for discussion Discuss the signs of attention-deficit hyperactivity disorder (ADHD) and learning disabilities (may be identified during this time in school) Upcoming milestones → Pubarche for males, abstract thinking, deductive reasoning, increasing connections with peer group
	SAFETY:	Revisit internet safety because with increasing independence and new handheld devices previous boundaries may need to be adjusted by the family. Parental control and apps can allow children some independent choices with parental oversight and restrictions to inappropriate content Bike helmets and traffic safety should be reviewed

11 & 12 Years

	NUTRITION
NATURAL FOODS:	Moderately active girls eat 1,800–2,000 calories/day, while boys eat between 2,000 and 2,200 calories/day[42] Ranges for food groups represent both female (low end of the range) and male (upper end of the range) recommendations 2 ½–3 cups+ of vegetables and 1 ½–2 cups+ of fruit daily
VITAMINS:	Vitamin and mineral intake should increase during puberty, so if diet lacking, a daily multivitamin may be necessary
IRON SOURCES:	5–6 oz of protein*; rarely a concern, as most adolescents in the United States eat twice as much protein as they need
GRAINS:	6–7 oz of grains^ with ½ coming from whole-grain sources
ADDED SUGAR/SALT:	Saturated fat and added sugar should be limited to <10% of daily calories; sodium should not exceed 1,900 mg/day
TEETH:	Permanent tooth eruption usually resumes until middle adolescence; time of highest rate of caries due to high carbohydrate diets, food choices, and hygiene practices; orthodontia may be needed; routine dental home evaluations recommended
DAIRY:	Recommended daily intake is 3 servings/day of reduced-fat milk or yogurt (8 oz) or cheese (1 ½ oz natural cheese)
	EXERCISE
CARDIOVASCULAR:	Chosen activity may meet daily cardiovascular and strengthening need (e.g., running is both cardiovascular and bone building)
STRENGTHENING:	Should engage in muscle strengthening and bone strengthening activities at least 3 days a week. Use of weight machines and handheld weights appropriate for tweens, as coordination, balance, and strength required to obtain benefits is present
	SLEEP
POSITION:	Ensure that tween is sleeping in a bed and not on a couch, chair, or the floor
QUANTITY:	10–12 hours/night; no naps; total: 10–12 hours Only about 15% of tweens or teens get recommended amount of sleep; likely due to a later evening melatonin release and a delayed drop in melatonin levels in the morning in combination with early school start times[57]
ROUTINE:	Hold over routines from elementary school continue to be helpful (warm bath or shower 1–1 ½ hours prior to bed, routine wake and sleep times that extend into the weekend, avoiding naps and "catch-up" sleep, etc.)
SLEEP HYGIENE:	No electronics near bedtime (currently 90% of teens use some electronic device within an hour of bedtime)[58]
	TRACKING
GROWTH:	Girls—Growth spurt (peak height velocity) occurs at ~11 ½ years old (usually 1 year after onset of puberty) and peak weight gain at ~12 years old; menarche typically occurs 2 years after onset of puberty or 1 year after peak height velocity Boys—Peak height velocity occurs at 13 ½ years old and it occurs 2 years after the onset of puberty. The peak weight gain occurs at the same time the peak height growth occurs

+½ cup = 1 serving
*1 oz = 1 oz of meat, poultry, or fish, ¼ cup of cooked dry beans, or 1 egg
^1 oz = 1 slice of bread, 1 cup of ready-to-eat cereal, ½ cup of cooked rice, pasta, or hot cereal

ADOLESCENTS

FAMILY & FRIENDS

FAMILY, INCLUDING SIBLINGS, PEER GROUP, & OUTSIDE SUPPORTS:	Ask about any recent changes in family (or peer group) structure or dynamic Get tween's opinion on household responsibilities—appropriate or overwhelming/interfering with school success Friends' parents Coaches, teachers, counselors, friends
ADJUSTMENT TO AGE OR STAGE:	Move toward more independence (Family counseling, if needed, for struggling parents and teens) Puberty (physical and emotional changes) Sleep, school, and activity schedules Homework demands
MONEY:	Patient may be able to earn own money from babysitting, lawn mowing, and so forth
SAFETY:	Seatbelt and helmet use Screening for illicit drugs begins at 11 years old, so candid questions about personal tobacco and marijuana use (cigarettes, e-cigs/vaping, chewing) are recommended, as well as discussing the health benefits of not using any of these substances

LEARNING

PHYSICAL DEVELOPMENT

PUBERTY:	Gangly and awkward; hands and feet grow prior to height growth in boys Increasing adiposity in females and decrease in males Changes in muscle distribution

COMMUNICATION/LANGUAGE DEVELOPMENT

VERBAL:	Increased ability to express self through speech, music, or art Adopts peer language and slang May appear introspective with limited conversations with adults

COGNITIVE/INTELLECTUAL DEVELOPMENT

INTELLIGENCE:	Move from concrete to inferential thinking Breadth and depth of knowledge increases	**PROBLEM-SOLVING:**	Approaches problems in a systematic manner Active problem-solving occurs during daydreaming

SOCIAL–EMOTIONAL DEVELOPMENT

CONNECTION:	Shift to more independence Same gender peers become support group with strong emotional feelings toward peers (love–hate relationships)	**SELF-REGULATION:**	Need for immediate gratification and lack of impulse control can lead to rudeness and risk-taking Pressure to conform may overrule better judgement Emotional lability (wide mood and behavior swings)

ADOLESCENTS

11 & 12 Years

YOUR TOOLS	
YOUR INTERVIEW:	Most of the interview should be focused on the tween, while balancing concerns and needs of parent. After discussing confidentiality rules, you may begin asking parent to step out of the room for one-on-one discussions with the tween to provide space for the tween to ask questions or answer more personal questions. Using the HEEADSS mnemonic allows the interview to move from questions that are less personal and less threatening, such as about home life and school, to those questions that may be more uncomfortable for the tween to discuss honestly, such as depression, drugs and sexuality.
YOUR OBSERVATIONS:	Aloof and reluctant to make eye contact, this patient may appear quite different from the last visit. Boys may appear awkward and gangly, while girls may have entered puberty with the subsequent redistribution of body proportions. In an attempt to control something in a world that feels completely out of their control, these kids experiment with their appearance, so a previously familiar kid now with a new hairstyle, hair color or fashion genre may sit on your exam table. When asked how things are going, you may get a one- or two-word response or you may learn new language/slang used by the patient's peer group. This is the patient's outward expression of the internal desire to fit in, yet be seen as a creative, independent person. Menarche, breast development and awkward body proportions are question that may come to the surface reluctantly.

PHYSICAL EXAM:		COMPLETE PHYSICAL EXAM WITH A SPECIFIC FOCUS ON	NORMAL FINDINGS YOU MIGHT SEE AT THIS AGE
	VITALS:	BMI BP percentile	BMI trending along growth curve BP percentile <90th percentile (www.mdcalc.com)
	EYES:	Assess internal eye structures, visual acuity	Visual acuity 20/25 or better
	NECK:	Palpate thyroid	Non-palpable thyroid
	MOUTH:	Inspect teeth, gums, and jaw	
	CHEST:	Auscultate for murmurs SMR	Pulmonary flow murmur Tanner Stage II–IV breasts
	MSK/NEURO:	Assess gait, stance, balance, and strength Evaluate for scoliosis in ♀	
	GENITALIA:	SMR, inguinal hernia	Tanner II–IV pubic hair (♀), menarche usually after Tanner IV pubic hair Tanner II genitalia with Tanner I pubic hair (♂)
	SKIN:	Signs of trauma/cutting, piercings, infections	Acne, increased sweating, body odor; hand drawn "tattoos" done with marker
	PSYCH:	Attention, focus, affect, overall dress and hair appearance	Seems to talk about some subjects and clam up about others; affect may be difficult to ascertain

ADOLESCENTS

11 & 12 Years

YOUR TOOLS		
SCREENINGS:	Auditory screening with 6,000 and 8,000 Hz high frequency (once between 11 and 14 years of age) Depression screening (12 years old) Tobacco, alcohol, and drug use screening (11 years old) Vision screening (12 years old)	*Optional based on history/risks/practice preference* Vision screening (11 years old)
IMMUNIZATIONS:	Tdap (if not done at 10 years old) MenACWY #1 HPV #1 (2nd dose can be given 6 months after the first) Influenza, if seasonally appropriate	

ANTICIPATORY GUIDANCE:	**Junior High Journey, Judgement, and Juggling Change (11–12 Years Old)** A large focus of the anticipatory guidance for this stage is around judgement and juggling	
	NUTRITION:	Food choices should include limited soda and sugar intake Reinforce need for foods rich in iron, calcium and vitamin D. If they aren't able to meet the 1,300 mg of calcium, 600 IU of vitamin D and 15 mg of iron, a supplement may be necessary[59]
	EXERCISE:	Emphasize need for 60 minutes of exercise daily Review importance of stretching and warm-up prior to strength and cardiovascular exercises Use of mouthguard in contact sports and discuss sport injury prevention
	SLEEP:	Quality sleep is important, and sleep should not be ignored when juggling multiple priorities Chronic sleep deprivation can lead to poor judgement, poor academic performance, and poor concentration[57]
	TRAJECTORY:	Discuss how difficult it can be to juggle new responsibilities, school demands, and social interests. Help tween articulate priorities and work through the barriers that are keeping them from reaching their goals Upcoming milestones → Increasing independence, abstract thinking, and continued pubertal changes
	SAFETY:	Providing a safe space for tweens/teens to talk about issues and concerns without judging them will help them feel supported Using one-on-one conversations, offering information to tweens/teens and allowing them to make their own conclusions is more effective than "lecturing" or "telling them what to do" Help families create a plan for discussing sexuality and pubertal developmental. Remind families and patients that puberty occurs in a predictable pattern, but the timing of that pattern falls on a spectrum. It is normal for breasts to bud anywhere from 9 to 13 years old and for menarche to occur anywhere from 10 ½ to 15 years old for girls

NUTRITION

NATURAL FOODS:	Moderately active girls require 2,000 calories/day, while boys need between 2,200 and 2,400 calories/day Ranges for food groups represent both female (low end of the range) and male (upper end of the range) recommendations 2 ½ - 3 cups[+] of vegetables and 2 cups[+] of fruits daily
VITAMINS:	Recommendation is 600 IU of vitamin D (equivalent to 8 servings of dairy or 4 oz of fish), 8–15 mg of iron (equivalent to 2–4 servings of iron-fortified cereal or iron-rich foods)[60] and 1,300 mg of calcium (equivalent to 4 ½ servings of dairy). Average intake of calcium is 500–1000 mg and only 13.7% of adolescent girls meet the iron recommendations[59]
IRON SOURCES:	5 ½–6 ½ oz/day of meat and beans*
GRAINS:	6–8 oz/day with ½ coming from whole-grain sources^
ADDED SUGAR/SALT:	Increasing intake of soda and "junk food" very common, but should recommend it be limited
TEETH:	Permanent tooth eruption is usually complete between 13 and 14 years old High rate of caries during teen years
DAIRY:	Recommended daily intake is 3 servings/day of reduced-fat milk, yogurt, or cheese

EXERCISE

CARDIOVASCULAR:	Chosen activity may meet daily cardiovascular and strengthening need (e.g., running is both cardiovascular and bone building)
STRENGTHENING:	Should engage in muscle strengthening and bone strengthening activities at least 3 days out of the week Use of weight machines and handheld weights OK

SLEEP

QUANTITY:	Recommendation is for 8–10 hours/night, but only 15% get this much[57] Naps rare, so teens taking 2–3 hour afternoon naps may have underlying sleep hygiene problem, depression, or school issues
ROUTINE:	Have a shift in sleep-wake cycle (staying up later and sleeping in)[57] Routine bedtime and waking time should extend into weekends with only about 60 minutes of extra sleep allowed
SLEEP SITE & SLEEP HYGIENE:	Make bedrooms "tech free" No electronics near bedtime

TRACKING

GROWTH:	Boys—Growth spurt (both height and weight) occurs ~13 ½ years old (usually 2 years after onset of puberty) Girls—Breast and pubic hair development complete by 14 ½ years old (average)
INTERVAL HISTORY:	Remember to update any interval illnesses and changes to the medical or family history

[+] ½ cup = 1 serving
*1 oz = 1 oz of meat, poultry, or fish, ¼ cup of cooked dry beans, or 1 egg
^1 oz = 1 slice of bread, 1 cup of ready-to-eat cereal, ½ cup of cooked rice, pasta, or hot cereal

ADOLESCENTS

FAMILY & FRIENDS

FAMILY, INCLUDING SIBLINGS, PEER GROUP, & OUTSIDE SUPPORTS:	Inquire about some form of privacy for the adolescent in the home Teen's opinion about family responsibilities—appropriate or overwhelming Ask about any recent changes in family or peer group structure/dynamic
	Coaches, teachers, peer group, another trusted adult
ADJUSTMENT TO AGE OR STAGE:	Move toward independence Puberty (physical and emotional changes) School/activity schedule and transition to high school Homework demands
MONEY:	Continue to ask about financial security/insecurity Money becomes more important to teens and social status may be linked to financial means Patient may be able to earn own money from babysitting, lawn mowing, and so forth
SAFETY:	Access to firearms and bullying Sexual coercion and dating violence, emotional abuse, or control characteristics Screening for illicit drugs should also include asking about personal tobacco and marijuana use (cigarettes, vaping, chewing)

LEARNING

PHYSICAL DEVELOPMENT

PUBERTY:	May develop body image concerns with changes in adipose tissue Increased interest in sexual anatomy, sexual experimentation, breast/penis size, menstruation, nocturnal emissions, and masturbation

COMMUNICATION/LANGUAGE DEVELOPMENT

VERBAL & WRITTEN:	Increased ability to express self through writing, speech, drawings Adopts peer language and slang	**NONVERBAL:**	Picks up on nonverbal cues more easily

COGNITIVE/INTELLECTUAL DEVELOPMENT

INTELLIGENCE:	Abstract thinking and creativity	**PROBLEM-SOLVING:**	Beginning to use deductive reasoning (if this, then that...)

SOCIAL–EMOTIONAL DEVELOPMENT

CONNECTION:	Creates new support group of same and opposite sex peers May be more introspective, feel disconnected from adults	**SELF-REGULATION:**	Poor impulse control leads to risk-taking Emotional lability (wide mood and behavior swings)

YOUR TOOLS

YOUR INTERVIEW:	Note: Many providers use the HEEADSS mnemonic when approaching the adolescent interview, so here are just a few modified HEEADSS questions:	
	HOME:	*Tell me about life at your house.*
	EDUCATION:	*What is your favorite subject in school?*
	EATING:	*What do you think makes for healthy eating? How close is this to your eating habits?*
	ACTIVITIES:	*Tell me about what you like to do outside of school.*
	DRUGS:	*Many patients tell me that they hear about people at school trying drugs and alcohol. What types of things have your classmates talked about trying? What are you tempted to experiment with? Why do you resist?*
	SEXUALITY:	*Are you attracted to boys, girls, or both? Do you feel tempted to experiment sexually? How do you resist?*
	SUICIDALITY:	*What do you see for your future?*
YOUR OBSERVATIONS:	This may be the first visit that the newly minted teenager comes back to the exam room unaccompanied. Not wanting to appear nervous, they may play it cool by trying to act like the whole process is boring and tired or they may just bury their heads in their smartphones pretending to be so popular and preoccupied that they can't be bothered by the rituals of the check-in. However, once you pop into the room, the phone is usually flipped over and laid next them on the exam table, keeping the crutch private, yet within reach. When asking questions, you may get short, staccato answers without much elaboration. When probed, answers may be punctuated with voice changes signaling a boy's early-to-mid pubertal state. The girls may have concerns about weight changes, irregular periods, and breast size, signaling her nearly complete pubertal transformation.	

		COMPLETE PHYSICAL EXAM WITH A SPECIFIC FOCUS ON	**NORMAL FINDINGS YOU MIGHT SEE AT THIS AGE**
PHYSICAL EXAM:	**VITALS:**	BP percentile	BP of <120/<80 mmHg
	NECK:	Palpating thyroid	Non-palpable thyroid
	MOUTH:	Inspect teeth and gums	Voice changes for males
	CHEST:	Auscultate for murmurs SMR breasts (♀)	SMR for females usually IV–V Physiologic gynecomastia in males[61]
	MSK/NEURO:	Assess gait, stance, balance, and strength Evaluate for scoliosis in ♂	
	GENITALIA:	SMR (♀ and ♂) Assess for direct or indirect hernias (♂)	SMR III–IV pubic hair, but IV–V genitalia (♂) Pearly penile papules; SMR III–V pubic hair (♀)
	SKIN:	Signs of self-harm, piercings, lesions/infections	Facial and back acne
	PSYCH:	Attention, affect, interaction with adults	

ADOLESCENTS			
	YOUR TOOLS		
SCREENINGS:	Auditory screening with 6,000 and 8,000 Hz high frequency (if not done at 11- or 12-year-old visit)[62] Depression screening (annually) Tobacco, alcohol, and drug use screening (annually)		*Optional based on history/risks/practice preference* Vision screening
IMMUNIZATIONS:	Usually none, if adolescent immunizations done at 10-, 11-, or 12-year-old visit Influenza annually, if seasonally appropriate		
ANTICIPATORY GUIDANCE:	**Knee-Jerk Reactions, Kindred Connections, and Keeping Up (13–14 Years Old)** The 2 Ks of this visit are keeping connected and knowledge		
	NUTRITION:	Diet should ensure adequate calcium and vitamin D intake, or you should recommend supplementation Remind patients to limit soda, junk food, and sugar intake Provide information on MyPlate app to help patient increase knowledge about nutrition requirements and to help decrease disordered eating, obesity	
	EXERCISE:	If not involved in organized sports, discuss safe strategies to get 60 minutes of exercise ≥4 times a week	
	SLEEP:	Parents should stay connected to kids around sleep routines and watch for excessive daytime sleepiness, napping, or poor concentration, all of which could signal an underlying mental health issue	
	TRAJECTORY:	School success is associated with a decrease in risky behaviors, so emphasizing the connection between school and success and positive efforts is key Talk with family about dance between teen and parent around responsibility and independence. A responsible teen earns more independence, while lack of responsibility typically means less freedom Knowledge and expectations to apply knowledge will continue to grow as teen enters high school Upcoming milestones → Increasing independence in decision making, improving executive function, understanding sexuality, and gaining resiliency skills	
	SAFETY:	Sexuality is a main focus of development, so begin to discuss pregnancy and sexually transmitted infection (STI) prevention Encourage families to watch for changes in mood, such as angry outbursts, more fighting with family members, depression, or anxiety, in their teen. Knowing how the teen is feeling, who they are hanging out with, and what they are thinking will give parents a keen sense of the teen's mental health Remind families that teens who have a connection to a trusted adult at home or at school are less likely to drop out of high school, usually have higher grades, tend to behave in a less risky manner, and are more apt to get help when faced with adversity.	

NUTRITION	
NATURAL FOODS:	Moderately active girls require 2,000 calories a day, while boys need between 2,600 and 2,800 calories a day Ranges for food groups represent both female (low end of the range) and male (upper end of the range) recommendations 2 ½–3 ½ cups[+] of vegetables/day and 2–2 ½ cups[+] of fruits
VITAMINS:	Adolescents tend to fall short of their daily quotas of calcium, iron, zinc, and vitamin D, so supplement if not getting from diet
IRON SOURCES:	5 ½–7 oz/day of meat and beans*
GRAINS:	6–10 oz/day with ½ coming from whole-grain sources^
ADDED SUGAR/SALT:	Limit sugar-sweetened beverages, energy drinks, and caffeinated boutique coffee drinks
TEETH:	Third molars (wisdom teeth) begin to erupt at ~17 to 18 years old Twice-daily brushing with fluorinated toothpaste and flossing once daily
DAIRY:	Recommended daily intake is three servings per day of reduced-fat milk, yogurt, or cheese, especially important for females who are laying down the bone that will carry them through maternity and lactation. Emphasize if on progesterone birth control
EXERCISE	
EXERCISE:	Weight-bearing exercise three times a week will serve to enhance bone strengthening, while 60 minutes of MVPA will help to reduce cardiovascular risks and can help to maintain a healthy weight
SLEEP	
POSITION:	Should be sleeping in a regular bed and not on the couch, in a chair, at a desk, or on the floor
QUANTITY:	Recommendation is for 8–10 hours each night, but only 15% get this much[57] Short (20–30 minute) naps may help keep normal sleep cycle at night
ROUTINE:	After a busy, hectic day, teens should build in time to unwind prior to bedtime. "Sleeping in" on the weekends should only extend an extra 1–2 hours longer than normal weekday routine[58]
SLEEP SITE & SLEEP HYGIENE:	Bedrooms should be "tech free," especially at bedtime Advisable to avoid caffeine, smoking, alcohol, and sleep aids at night Bed should be used only for sleeping—not as a study pod, a reading nook, or a gaming chair
TRACKING	
GROWTH:	Growth slows after the peak height velocity (males) and peak weight velocity (females) When close to adult stature, growth decelerates to ~1 cm/year
INTERVAL HISTORY:	Changes to the health history, family history, social history, or past medical history should be captured

[+]½ cup = 1 serving
*1 oz = 1 oz of meat, poultry, or fish, ¼ cup of cooked dry beans, or 1 egg
^1 oz = 1 slice of bread, 1 cup of ready-to-eat cereal, ½ cup of cooked rice, pasta, or hot cereal

ADOLESCENTS

FAMILY & FRIENDS			
Family, Including Siblings, Peer Group, & Outside Supports:	Where is teen living? Assess for homelessness or couch surfing What are the rules/expectations/boundaries for teen around household help, homework, extracurricular activities, curfew, dress, dating, and so forth?		
	Do patient's parents know the parents of teen's friends? Other support such as coaches, teachers, counselors, friends		
Adjustment to Age or Stage:	Increased independence with decreased family involvement Emotional lability (family counseling can be offered if disruptive to family dynamic) Learning to drive Sexual feelings and relationships		
Money:	May start working after school or on weekends to earn own money (or may be earning money to help support family finances)		
Safety:	Home, neighborhood, and school safety Interpersonal violence or sexual coercion Ask about personal tobacco, alcohol, and drug exposures and discuss health benefits of not engaging in any substance use		
LEARNING			
Physical Development			
Post-Puberty:	May appear older than developmental age		
Communication/Language Development			
Verbal & Written:	May be opinionated about political and philosophical viewpoints May have a "you don't understand" attitude toward parents		
Cognitive/Intellectual Development			
Intelligence:	Abstract thinking Introspection	**Problem-Solving:**	Improving executive function Beginning to make judgments using sound reasoning, but still resorts to emotional decisions
Social–Emotional Development			
Connection:	Possible labile relationship with parents Increasing interest in romantic relationships	**Self-Regulation:**	Still impulsive, but some logic in decision-making Begins demonstrating resiliency when faced with life stressors Begins to become comfortable with one's sexuality and is learning to express/control sexual drives

ADOLESCENTS

YOUR TOOLS		
YOUR INTERVIEW:	Note: Many providers use the HEEADSS mnemonic when approaching the adolescent interview, so here are just a few modified HEEADSS questions:	
	HOME:	*Who lives with you? How do you get along with everyone in the house?*
	EDUCATION:	*What is the most enjoyable thing about school? What is the most stressful thing about school?*
	EATING:	*Tell me what you like about your body and what you would change if you could.*
	ACTIVITIES:	*How much exercise do you get each day (or week)?*
	DRUGS:	*What do you know about the risks of drinking alcohol? smoking? huffing? taking prescription drugs? using other drugs, like marijuana, ecstasy or heroin?*
	SEXUALITY:	*One of the big tasks now that you are completing puberty is to become comfortable with your sexuality. What does that make you think, when I say that?* *Would you like to become a parent in the next year? When would it be a good time to become a parent?*
	SAFETY:	*Tell me what you do to deal with stress at school or in your personal life.*
YOUR OBSERVATIONS:	Slightly more self-confident, the middle adolescent may feel more at ease with asking and answering some of the more sensitive topics during the interview. They will likely make more eye contact, have a more adult outward appearance and demeanor, and use clothing and appearance to set themselves apart from others. With many having obtained their licenses, they may drive to the appointment alone and you may not have an opportunity to engage with their parents as you have in the past. Most will have completed puberty and much of the visit will focus on risk reduction counseling, future planning and ensuring proper scaffolding for social, emotional and problem-solving support.	

PHYSICAL EXAM:		COMPLETE PHYSICAL EXAM WITH A SPECIFIC FOCUS ON	NORMAL FINDINGS YOU MIGHT SEE AT THIS AGE
	VITALS:	BP percentile	BP of <120/<80 mmHg
	NECK:	Palpate thyroid	
	CHEST:	Auscultate for murmurs Assess breast tissue	Physiologic gynecomastia may persist for some boys[61]
	MSK/NEURO:	Assess gait, stance, balance, and strength Evaluate for scoliosis in ♂	
	GENITALIA:	SMR (♀ and ♂) Assess for direct or indirect hernias (♂)	SMR V pubic hair and genitalia (♂)[63] SMR V pubic hair (♀)[63]
	SKIN:	Signs of self-harm, piercings, infections, lesions	Facial and back acne
	PSYCH:	Assess thinking, logic/reasoning, affect/mood	

<table>
<tr><td colspan="3" align="center">YOUR TOOLS</td></tr>
<tr>
<td rowspan="1">SCREENINGS:</td>
<td>Auditory screening with 6,000 and 8,000 Hz high frequency (once between 15 and 17 years old and once between 18 and 21 years old)[62]
Depression screening (annually)
Tobacco, alcohol, and drug use screening (annually)
Universal HIV screening (at ≥15 years old)
Vision screening (at 15 years old)</td>
<td>Optional based on history/risks/practice preference
If sexually active, baseline screening for Neisseria gonorrhoeae, Chlamydia trachomatis, Trichomonas vaginalis, HIV, Hepatitis B, and syphilis[64]
Vision screening at 16, 17, and 18 years old</td>
</tr>
<tr>
<td>IMMUNIZATIONS:</td>
<td colspan="2">MenACWY #2 (at 16 years old)
MenB (16–18 years old)
HPV (3 dose series, if not done previous)
Influenza, annually, if seasonally appropriate</td>
</tr>
<tr>
<td rowspan="6">ANTICIPATORY GUIDANCE:</td>
<td colspan="2" align="center">Love, Licenses, and Life After High School (15–18 Years Old)
Anticipatory guidance centers on 4 Ls—lowering risk, long-term goals, long-acting reversible contraceptives, and licenses</td>
</tr>
<tr>
<td>NUTRITION:</td>
<td>Encourage healthy food choices and review dangers of skipping meals
Provide evidence-based information on weight loss, if necessary</td>
</tr>
<tr>
<td>EXERCISE:</td>
<td>Encourage 60 minutes of exercise the majority of the days of the week</td>
</tr>
<tr>
<td>SLEEP:</td>
<td>Review importance of 8–9 hours of sleep nightly and sleep hygiene</td>
</tr>
<tr>
<td>TRAJECTORY:</td>
<td>Use teen's long-term goals as a springboard to discuss choices and behaviors that can either help or hurt the teen's ability to reach these goals. Using this approach may allow the teen to open himself up to more discussions
Older teens should begin discussing post–high school plans and how current academics and activities are helping to move toward the goals
Depending on your practice setting and the patient's preference, you may want to begin discussing a transition of care to a college health center, family medicine, or internal medicine provider for ongoing care</td>
</tr>
<tr>
<td>SAFETY:</td>
<td>Educate newly licensed teens on risks of driving at night and texting and driving, as motor vehicle accidents are one of the leading causes of death in this age group[65]
Risk reduction strategies that focus on injury, misuse of prescription drugs, drug and alcohol use, and peer pressure are important
High-risk sexual behaviors can have an impact on long-term goals, so provide reliable, straightforward information on safe sex practices, coercion, STIs, and unintended pregnancy
Provide education on abstinence, family planning options, and long-acting reversible contraceptives (LARCs), when appropriate</td>
</tr>
</table>

NUTRITION	
NATURAL FOODS:	Proper sports nutrition can help promote optimal performance, growth, body composition, and immunity in young athletes[66] Sport-specific nutrition knowledge is inadequate for many coaches, student athletes, and parents[67] Athletes require balanced diets and higher calorie intakes with focus on whole grains and iron-rich proteins[42] Student athletes don't generally ask providers for advice about supplement use, so providers should ask; not recommended for kids/teens[68]
VITAMINS:	Athletes need adequate calcium and vitamin D for bone development Vitamin C, magnesium, and zinc help boost the immune system[69,70]
IRON SOURCES:	Essential for carrying oxygen to muscles, so need adequate lean meat, fish, and poultry Other sources may include green leafy vegetables and iron-fortified cereals
GRAINS:	Whole-grains digest slowly and provide longer-lasting energy
ADDED SUGAR/SALT:	Ask about "energy" drinks that contain high levels of sugar and caffeine; avoid sports drinks that contain high sugar content
TEETH:	Should have a mouth guard if participating in contact sports with risk of collision/injury
DAIRY:	The recommended 3 cups/day of dairy is important for the protein and the calcium and vitamin D
EXERCISE	
AEROBIC:	Couple aerobic conditioning with resistance training for a more complete work-out Should exercise all muscle groups, including the core, and perform exercises at full ROM
STRENGTH TRAINING:	Children and teens should begin with low-resistance training and once athlete can do 2–3 sets of 8–15 reps with proper form, then OK to add in small increments of weight[53] Strength training should be incorporated 2–3 times per week, as > 4 times a week doesn't allow for adequate recovery[71]
SLEEP	
SECRET TO SUCCESS:	Without appropriate amounts of sleep, young athletes: • Are more likely to sustain an injury • Take longer to recover from sports-related concussion • Have more difficulty learning a new skill or improving skills • Perform poorer academically • Are unable to perform at maximum potential[72]
TIMING	
WHEN TO PERFORM:	A pre-participation exam (PPE) should ideally be performed 4–6 weeks prior to the start of the athletic season/activity to allow time for conditioning and rehabilitation of injuries, referrals, and rechecks

ADOLESCENTS

FACTS	
PERSONAL HISTORY IMPORTANT TO THE PPE:	Any specific conditions in the past medical history that could affect participation Hospitalizations Surgeries, including orthopedic surgeries Current medications Allergies Menstrual patterns (to investigate female athlete triad)
SPORT-SPECIFIC HISTORY IMPORTANT TO THE PPE:	Previous restrictions or withholdings from participating in a sport for medical reason Dental trauma Dermatologic issues (MRSA infections, herpes infections, unhealing sores) Cardiopulmonary issues (chest pain with exercise, heart palpitations, feeling faint or having passed out with exercise, excessive shortness of breath or fatigue with exercise) Neurologic issues ("burners" or "stingers," mild traumatic brain injury/concussion, headaches with exercise) Orthopedic problems (sprains, fractures, dislocations, orthopedic device use, bone/muscle/joint pain, back or neck injuries)
FAMILY HISTORY IMPORTANT TO THE PPE:	Anyone in the family with: • Asthma • Diabetes • High BP/hypertension • Heart problems, specifically hypertrophic or dilated cardiomyopathy, arrhythmias, long or short QT syndrome, Brugada syndrome, a pacemaker, implanted defibrillator • Marfan syndrome • Near drowning episode • Unexpected death before the age of 50 • Unexplained fainting or seizures

LEVEL OF CONTACT*					
CONTACT:	Basketball Cheerleading Field and ice hockey Football Soccer Wrestling	**LIMITED-CONTACT:**	Baseball Field events (high jump, pole vault) Skiing Skating Softball Volleyball	**NON-CONTACT:**	Cross country Golf Swimming Tennis Track

*Please check your local county and state regulations, as these are only a few examples.

Pre-Participation Exam

ADOLESCENTS

Pre-Participation Exam

YOUR TOOLS		
	PHYSICAL EXAM WITH A SPECIFIC FOCUS ON	**CONCERNING FINDINGS INCLUDE[73,74]**
PHYSICAL EXAM:	**VITALS:** Pulse, BP, height, weight, BMI	High BP (>130/80 or ≥95th percentile if younger than 13 years) → Needs further evaluation/possible treatment
	GENERAL: Marfan stigmata	Long limbs relative to trunk, arachnodactyly, pectus deformity could indicate Marfan's syndrome, which carries a risk of aortic dissection → Referral to cardiology for evaluation and clearance
	SKIN: Lesions/rashes	Herpes simplex, impetigo, molluscum, scabies, tinea corporis, or varicella should be considered contagious → Treat prior to clearance
	HEAD: Position	A tilt to one side could indicate cervical muscle strain, C-spine injury, or trapezius strain
	EYES: Visual acuity	Corrected vision of 20/40 or worse requires eye protection and evaluation by eye specialist
	EARS: Deformities	Cauliflower ear likely indicates previous trauma without use of proper head gear
	MOUTH: Lip lesions Braces	Lesions consistent with herpes or impetigo indicate a contagious infection → Treatment needed prior to return to sports
	NECK: ROM, strength and point tenderness	Loss of flexion, lateral bending, and/or rotation concerning for previous neck injury
	CARDIO/ PULMONARY: 1. Murmurs, clicks, rubs, gallops 2. Point of maximal impulse (PMI) 3. Femoral pulses and radial-femoral delay 4. Lungs	1. A crescendo-decrescendo murmur that increases in intensity with Valsalva or gets softer with squatting is concerning for hypertrophic obstructive cardiomyopathy 2. Displaced PMI is concerning for cardiomegaly 3. A weak or non-palpable femoral pulse or a delay between radial and femoral pulse are concerning for coarctation of aorta 4. Wheezes after activity could indicate exercise-induced asthma
	ABDOMEN: Organomegaly	
	GENITALIA: Presence of two testicles Direct or indirect hernia (♂)	

<table>
<tr><td rowspan="2" style="writing-mode:vertical">ADOLESCENTS</td><td colspan="3" align="center">YOUR TOOLS</td><td rowspan="2" style="writing-mode:vertical">Pre-Participation Exam</td></tr>
<tr><td colspan="2" align="center">PHYSICAL EXAM WITH A SPECIFIC FOCUS ON</td><td align="center">CONCERNING FINDINGS INCLUDE[73,74]</td></tr>
</table>

	PHYSICAL EXAM WITH A SPECIFIC FOCUS ON	CONCERNING FINDINGS INCLUDE[73,74]
SHOULDER:	• Asymmetry or bony prominences • ROM and joint stability (evaluate abduction with straight arm abduction to overhead position and abduction and external rotation by having athlete put hands at base of skull and pull elbows back as far as possible) • Strength (check with resisted shoulder shrug; resisted flexion and abduction)	• Enlarged acromioclavicular or sternoclavicular joint may indicate previous separation, but if nontender → No concern • Asymmetric shoulder height could indicate trapezius or paraspinous strain/spasm, limb length discrepancy, or scoliosis • Asymmetric shoulder elevation or inability to fully abduct arms is worrisome for weakness or instability • Hesitancy to perform hands behind head maneuver may indicate incompletely rehabilitated glenohumeral joint subluxation • Weakness when shrugging is concerning for trapezius injury • Weakness with resisted abduction indicates deltoid injury
ELBOW:	ROM (athlete puts arms at the sides, extends and flexes the elbow, then at a 90° elbow position pronates/supinates)	Incomplete extension, flexion, supination, or pronation may signal an old injury, dislocation, or fracture
HANDS:	ROM and deformities (have athlete spread fingers, then make a fist)	A protruding knuckle, crooked finger, decreased flexion, or swollen finger may indicate old fractures or sprains
BACK:	• Scoliosis (Adam's forward-bend test) • Midline tenderness • Iliac crest heights	• Midline lumbar pain in extension may indicate spondylolysis • Asymmetric iliac crests are concerning for scoliosis, leg length discrepancy, pelvic rotation, or lumbar muscle spasm
KNEE & HIP:	• Swelling, redness • Strength and ROM (duck walk) • Knee and hip position upon landing after a jump for female athletes	• Prominent, tender tibial tuberosity indicates Osgood-Schlatter • Inability to duck walk may point to muscle weakness • Pain with duck walk indicates a meniscal tear • Landing with valgus positioning on patella and internal rotation of the hip signals female athlete is at risk for an ACL injury[75]
CALF & ANKLE:	• Ankle stability (ask athlete to hop x 5 on each foot) • Muscle atrophy (view calves while athlete raises up on toes)	• Inability to hop without pain or instability is concerning for an undiagnosed or incompletely rehabilitated ankle or foot injury • Calf asymmetry may represent an Achilles injury or a unrehabilitated ankle injury

(Row label for whole table: **PHYSICAL EXAM:**)

YOUR TOOLS		
SCREENINGS:	Auditory screening, if available Vision screening	
IMMUNIZATIONS:	Time to provide any catch-up immunizations	
ANTICIPATORY GUIDANCE:	**Move It, Move It…Making Sure Kids Are Safe to Participate in Athletics** The main anticipatory guidance principles for the pre-participation exam are the 3 Ms—musculoskeletal protection, meals, and meeting academic expectations	
	NUTRITION:	Ensure that the athlete is consuming adequate calories for anticipated activities with appropriate protein and carbohydrate ratios[68] Eat a light snack or meal 2–4 hours before game/competition and stop eating at least 1 hour before the event to save energy (digestion requires energy, which takes away from energy available for activity) Young athletes should be advised to avoid meal replacements and unproven supplements[68] Athletes should avoid carbonated drinks or juice while competing
	EXERCISE:	Rest at least once a week and take at least 1 month off of training during the year Athlete should hydrate before, during, and after exercise. Recommend drinking 16 oz of water 2 hours prior to and 8 oz 15 minutes prior to activity, 6–8 oz every 15 minutes during, and 24 oz after activity[68]
	SLEEP:	Sleep routines and adequate sleep are essential for top performance in athletics and in school Need more sleep for healing injuries and restoration
	TIMING:	Encourage athletes to begin training 6–8 weeks prior to a sport season, if possible Remind athletes and families that school/academics should be prioritized before sports participation Meeting academic expectations may need to become top priority if student athlete becomes ineligible to participate due to grades
	SAFETY:	Review conditioning strategies for male and female athletes with particular attention to most common injuries based on sport-specific injury profiles (e.g., ACL tears and concussions in female athletes, overuse injuries and "cutting weight" in male athletes) Encourage dynamic stretching before exercise, as it increases blood flow to the muscles, helps with joint flexibility, and improves ROM, all of which help prevent injury[76] Progressive strengthening of core and lower extremities, jump training, and feedback on jump technique can reduce ACL injuries by 75%[77]

REFERENCES

1. Clinical Growth Charts. Centers for Disease Control and Prevention National Center of Health Statistics website. June 16, 2017. https://www.cdc.gov/growthcharts/clinical_charts.htm.

2. Weintraub B. Growth. *Pediatr Rev.* 2010;32(9):404–406.

3. Phillips SM, Shulman RJ. Measurement of growth in children. In: Motil K, ed. *UpToDate.* UpToDate, Inc.; October 29, 2020.

4. Braun LR, Marino R. Disorders of growth and stature. *Pediatr Rev.* 2017;38(7):293–302.

5. Spivak H, Sege R, Flanigan E, Licenziato V, eds. *Connected Kids: Safe, Strong, Secure Clinical Guide.* American Academy of Pediatrics; 2006.

6. O'Keefe L. Identifying food insecurity: Two-question screening tool has 97% sensitivity. *AAP News.* October 23, 2015. https://www.aappublications.org/content/early/2015/10/23/aapnews.20151023-1.

7. Rabin RF, Jennings JM, Campbell JC, Bair-Merritt M. Intimate partner violence screening tools. *Am J Prev Med.* 2009;36(5):439–445.

8. Daniels SR, Benuck I, Christakis DA, et al. In: Services USDoHaH, ed. *National Heart, Lung, and Blood Institute Expert Panel on Integrated Guidelines for Cardiovascular Health and Risk Reduction in Children and Adolescents—Full Report.* National Institutes of Health; October 2012. NIH Publication No. 12-7486.

9. Deoni SCL, Mercure E, Blasi A, et al. Mapping infant brain myelination with magnetic resonance imaging. *J Neurosci.* January 2011;31(2):784–791.

10. Lawrence RA, Lawrence RM. *Breastfeeding: A Guide for the Medical Profession.* 7th ed. Elsevier|Mosby; 2011.

11. Eidelman AI, Schanler RJ. Breastfeeding and the use of human milk. *Pediatrics.* March 2012;129(3):e827–e841.

12. Li R, Fein SB, Chen J, Grummer-Strawn LM. Why mothers stop breastfeeding: Mothers' self-reported reasons for stopping during the first year. *Pediatrics.* 2008;122:S69–S76.

13. Feldman-Winter L. *Improving Our Approach: Better Conversations about Breastfeeding.* NICHQ; November 7, 2018.

14. American Academy of Pediatrics Committee on Practice and Ambulatory Medicine BFPSW. 2020 Recommendations for preventive pediatric health care. 2020.

15. Immunization schedules for health care providers. Centers for Disease Control and Prevention. February 3, 2020. https://www.cdc.gov/vaccines/schedules/.

16. Wagner CL, Greer FR, American Academy of Pediatrics Section on Breastfeeding, American Academy of Pediatrics Committee on Nutrition. Prevention of rickets and vitamin D deficiency in infants, children, and adolescents. *Pediatrics.* November 2008;122(5):1142–1152.

17. Riordan J, Wambach K. *Breastfeeding and Human Lactation.* 4th ed. Jones and Bartlett Publishers; 2010.

18. AAP Task Force on Sudden Infant Death Syndrome. SIDS and other sleep-related infant deaths: Updated 2016 recommendations for a safe infant sleeping environment. *Pediatrics.* November 2016;138(5):e2016–e2938.

19. Flaherman VJ, Schaefer EW, Kuzniewicz MW, et al. Early weight loss nomograms for exclusively breastfed newborns. *Pediatrics.* January 2015;35(1):e16–e23.

20. Age-appropriate vision milestones. Stanford children's health. 2020. https://www.stanfordchildrens.org/en/topic/default?id=age-appropriate-vision-milestones-90-P02305.

21. Drutz JE. The pediatric physical examination: HEENT. In: Duryea T, ed. *UpToDate*. UpToDate Inc; July 8, 2019. https://www.uptodate.com/contents/the-pediatric-physical-examination-heent.

22. Marcdante KJ, Kliegman RM. Assessment of the mother, fetus, and newborn. In: Marcdante KJ, Kliegman RM, eds. *Nelson Essentials of Pediatrics*. 8th ed. Elsevier, Inc.; 2019:217–235.

23. McKee-Garrett TM. Assessment of the newborn infant. In: Martin RM, Duryea TK, eds. *UpToDate*. UpToDate, Inc.; June 29, 2020. https://www.uptodate.com/contents/assessment-of-the-newborn-infant.

24. Mathes E, Howard RM. Vesicular, pustular, and bullous lesions in the newborn and infant. In: Levy M, Edwards MS, eds. *UpToDate*. UpToDate Inc; December 3, 2018. https://www.uptodate.com/contents/vesicular-pustular-and-bullous-lesions-in-the-newborn-and-infant.

25. Saunders NR. Innocent heart murmurs in children: Taking a diagnostic approach. *Can Fam Physician*. 1995;41:1507–1512.

26. Keys C, Heloury Y. Retractile testes: A review of the current literature. *J Pediatr Urol*. 2012;8:2–6.

27. Barr M. What is the period of PURPLE crying? The period of PURPLE crying website. http://purplecrying.info/what-is-the-period-of-purple-crying.php. Accessed August 19, 2020.

28. Holt KA, ed. *Bright Futures: Nutrition and Pocket Guide*. 3rd ed. American Academy of Pediatrics; 2011.

29. Coats DK. Vision screening and assessment in infants and children. In: Paysse E, Olitsky, SE, eds. *UpToDate*. UpToDate, Inc; November 27, 2018. https://www.uptodate.com/contents/vision-screening-and-assessment-in-infants-and-children.

30. Mayo Clinic Staff. Iron deficiency in children: Prevention tips for parents. December 10, 2019. Mayo Clinic.org. Healthy Lifestyle: Children's Health Web site. https://www.mayoclinic.org/healthy-lifestyle/childrens-health/in-depth/iron-deficiency/art-20045634.

31. Centers for Disease Control and Prevention. Recommendations to prevent and control iron deficiency in the United States. *MMWR*. 1998;47(RR-3):1–29.

32. Bonyata K. Is iron supplementation necessary? KellyMom website. May 21, 2018. https://kellymom.com/nutrition/vitamins/iron/.

33. Clark MB, Slayton RL, Section on Oral Health. Fluoride use in caries prevention in the primary care setting. *Pediatrics*. 2014;134(3):626–633.

34. Ziegler EE. Adverse effects of cow's milk in infants. *Nestle Nutr Workshop Ser Pediatr Program*. 2007;60:185–199.

35. Sleep Foundation. When do babies sleep through the night? Sleep Foundation: A OneCare Media Company. December 17, 2020. https://www.sleepfoundation.org/baby-sleep/when-do-babies-sleep-through-night.

36. American Academy of Pediatrics Subcommittee on Management of Acute Otitis Media. Diagnosis and management of acute otitis media. *Pediatrics*. 2004;113(5):1451–1465.

37. ADA Division of Communications. Tooth eruption: The primary teeth. *J Am Dental Assn*. November 2005;136:1619.

38. Heyman MB, Abrams SA, Section on Gastroenterology, Hepatology, and Nutrition, Committee On Nutrition. Fruit juice in infants, children and adolescents: Current recommendations. *Pediatrics*. June 2017;139(6):e20170967.

39. Children's Dental Health Project. AAP recommends earlier use of toothpaste. September 2, 2014. Children's Dental Health Project: Teeth Matter. https://www.cdhp.org/blog/307-aap-recommends-earlier-use-of-toothpaste.

40. American Academy of Pediatric Dentistry. Parent: Frequently Asked Questions (FAQ). 2021. https://www.aapd.org/resources/parent/faq/.

41. Gavin ML. Growth and your 1- to 2-year-old. KidsHealth from Nemours: For Parents. June 2019. https://kidshealth.org/en/parents/grow12yr.html.

42. 2020 Dietary Guidelines Advisory Committee and Food Pattern Modeling Team. *Food Pattern Modeling: Ages 2 Years and Older.* U.S. Department of Agriculture; 2020.

43. Flossing and Children. Lucile Packard Children's Hospital Stanford. 2021. https://www.stanfordchildrens.org/en/topic/default?id=%20 flossing-and-children-90-P01852.

44. Evans A. *Pocket Podiatry: Paediatrics.* Churchill Livingstone-Elsevier; 2010.

45. Kennedy E. My golden rule to building healthy toddler meals and snacks. My Little Eater website. https://mylittleeater.com/my-golden -rule-to-building-healthy-toddler-meals-and-snacks/. Accessed August 18, 2020.

46. Center for Nutrition Policy and Promotion. *MyPlate Plan—Food Group Amounts for 1,200 Calories a Day.* United States Department of Agriculture; January 2016.

47. Pacheco D. Night terrors. Sleep Foundation: A OneCare Media Company. October 2, 2020. https://www.sleepfoundation.org/night-terrors.

48. Wiseman J. Sleep strategies for kids. Sleep Foundation: A OneCare Media Company. September 24, 2020. https://www.sleepfoundation .org/children-and-sleep/sleep-strategies-kids.

49. Harding EC, Franks NP, Wisden W. The temperature dependence of sleep. *Front Neurosci.* 2019;13:336.

50. Cooke DA, Divall SA, Radovick S. Normal and aberrant growth in children. In: Melmed S, Polonsky KS, Larsen PR, Kronenberg HM, eds. *Williams Textbook of Endocrinology*. 13th ed. Elsevier; 2016:964–1073.

51. Gavin ML. Growth and your 6- to 12-year-old. KidsHealth from Nemours: For Parents. June 2019. https://kidshealth.org/en/parents/ growth-6-12.html.

52. Faigenbaum AD, Bruno LE. A fundamental approach for treating pediatric dynapenia in kids. *ACSM's Health Fit J.* July/August 2017;2(4):18–24.

53. Stricker PR, Faigenbaum AD, McCambridge TM. Resistance training for children and adolescents. *Pediatrics.* June 2020;145(6): e20201011.

54. Davies D. *Child Development: A Practitioner's Guide.* 3rd ed. Guilford Press; 2011.

55. Council on Sports Medicine and Fitness. Strength training by children and adolescents. *Pediatrics.* April 2008;121(4):835–840.

56. U.S. Department of Health and Human Services. *Physical Activity Guidelines for Americans*. 2nd ed. U.S. Department of Health and Human Services; 2018.

57. Suni E. Teens and sleep. Sleep Foundation: A OneCare Media Company. August 5, 2020. https://www.sleepfoundation.org/articles/ teens-and-sleep.

58. Sleep and Teens. UCLA Health.org. Patient Education website. https:// www.uclahealth.org/sleepcenter/sleep-and-teens. Accessed November 13, 2020.

59. Demory-Luce D, Motil KJ. Adolescent eating habits. In: Middlemen A, ed. *UpToDate.* UpToDate, Inc; April 8, 2020. https://www.uptodate .com/contents/adolescent-eating-habits.

60. Powers JM. Iron requirements and iron deficiency in adolescents. In: Abrams S, Motil KJ, Mahoney DH, Blake D, eds. *UpTo Date.* UpToDate, Inc; March 25, 2020. https://www.uptodate.com/ contents/iron-requirements-and-iron-deficiency-in-adolescents.

61. Lemaine V, Cayci C, Simmons PS, Petty P. Gynecomastia in adolescent males. *Semin Plast Surg.* February 2013;27(1):56–61.

62. Shaw JF, Jr., Shaw JS, Duncan PM, eds. *Bright Futures: Guidelines for Health Supervision of Infants, Children, and Adolescents.* 4th ed. American Academy of Pediatrics; 2017.

63. Neinstein LS. *Adolescent Health Care: A Practical Guide.* Lippincott Williams & Wilkins; 2002.

64. American Academy of Pediatrics Committee on Infectious Diseases. Sexually transmitted infections in adolescents and children. In: Kimberlin D, ed. *Red Book: 2018–2021 Report of the Committee on Infectious Diseases.* 31st ed. American Academy of Pediatrics; 2018.

65. Curtin SC, Heron M, Minino AM, Warner, M. *Recent Increases in Injury Mortality Among Children and Adolescents aged 10–19 Years in the United States: 1999–2016.* U.S. Department of Health and Human Services, Centers for Disease Control and Prevention National Center for Health Statistics; June 1 2018.

66. Rodriguez NR, Di Marco NM, Langley S. American College of Sports Medicine position stand. Nutrition and athletic performance. *Med Sci Sports Exerc.* 2009;41(3):709–731.

67. Thomas M, Nelson TF, Harwood, E, Neumark-Sztainer D. Exploring parent perceptions of the food environment in youth sports. *J Nutr Educ Behav.* 2011;44(4):365–371.

68. Nutrition and Supplement Use. American academy of pediatrics. March 12, 2012. https://www.healthychildren.org/English/healthy-living/ nutrition/Pages/Nutrition-and-Supplement-Use.aspx.

69. Gavin ML. Minerals. KidsHealth from Nemours: For Kids. August 2015. https://kidshealth.org/en/kids/minerals.html.

70. Gavin ML. Vitamins. KidsHealth from Nemours: For Kids. July 2014. https://kidshealth.org/en/kids/vitamin.html.

71. Faigenbaum AD, Kraemer WJ, Blimkie CJR, et al. Youth resistance training: Updated position statement paper from the national strength and conditioning association. *J Strength Cond Res.* 2009;23: S60–S79.

72. Sleep Foundation. Do student athletes need extra sleep? Sleep Foundation: A OneCare Media Company. https://www.sleepfoundation .org/articles/do-student-athletes-need-extra-sleep.

73. Mirabelli MH, Devine MJ. The preparticipation sports evaluation. *Am Fam Physician.* September 2015;92(5):371–376.

74. Hergenroeder AC. Sports participation in children and adolescents: The preparticipation physical evaluation. In: Chorley J, Triedman JK, eds. *UpToDate.* UpToDate, Inc; January 6, 2020. https://www.uptodate. com/contents/sports-participation-in-children-and-adolescents-the -preparticipation-physical-evaluation.

75. Dharamsi A, Labella CR. Prevention of ACL injuries in adolescent female athletes. *Contemporary Pediatrics.* 2013. https://www. contemporarypediatrics.com/view/prevention-acl-injuries-adolescent -female-athletes.

76. Gavin ML. Stretching. KidsHealth from Nemours: For Teens. September 2018. TeensHealth from Nemours Web site. https://kidshealth.org/en/ teens/stretching.html.

77. Padua DA, DiStefano LJ, et al. National athletic trainers' association position statement: Prevention of anterior cruciate ligament injury. *J Athl Train.* 2018;53(1):5–19.

AAP	American Academy of Pediatrics
ACEs	adverse childhood events
ACIP	Advisory Committee on Immunization Practices
ACL	anterior cruciate ligament
ADHD	attention-deficit hyperactivity disorder
AFOSF	anterior fontanelle is open, soft, and flat
ASQ®	Ages and Stages Questionnaires®
ATNR	asymmetrical tonic neck reflex
BF	breastfeeding
BMI	body mass index
BP	blood pressure
CDC	Centers for Disease Control and Prevention
CHIP	Children's Health Insurance Program
CPR	cardiopulmonary resuscitation
CRAFFT	Car, Relax, Alone, Forget, Friends, Trouble
CTA	clear to auscultation
CV	cardiovascular
DTaP	diphtheria, tetanus, and acellular pertussis
ECE	early childhood education
EHRs	electronic health records
EOM(I)	extraocular movements (intact)
EPDS	Edinburgh Postnatal Depression Scale
FAMS	family and siblings, adjustment to the age or stage, monetary concerns, safety
FLY	family support, learned skills, your tools
FP	femoral pulse
HC	head circumference
HEEADSS(S)	adolescent interview mnemonic, which includes asking about home, education/employment, eating, activities, drugs, sexuality, suicidality, and sometimes safety
HepA	hepatitis A
HepB	hepatitis B
Hib	*Haemophilus influenzae* type b
HIV	human immunodeficiency virus
HPV	human papillomavirus
HS	high school
HSM	hepatosplenomegaly
IEP	individualized education program
IIV	inactivated influenza vaccine
IPV	interpersonal violence or intimate partner violence or inactivated poliovirus
LARCs	long-acting reversible contraceptives
LD	learning disability
LE	lower extremity
M-CHAT™	Modified Checklist for Autism in Toddlers™
MenACWY	meningococcal serogroup A, C, W, Y
MenB	meningococcal serogroup B
MMR	measles, mumps, and rubella
MRSA	methicillin-resistant *Staphylococcus aureus*
MSK	musculoskeletal
MV	multivitamin

MVPA	moderate to vigorous physical activity
NaVIGATeD	natural foods, vitamins, iron sources, grains, added sugar and salt, teeth, dairy
NC/AT	normocephalic and atraumatic
NEST	nutrition, elimination or exercise, sleep, tracking
O/B	Ortolani and Barlow maneuvers
O/P	oropharynx
OCP	oral contraceptive pills
PCV13	pneumococcal vaccine
PE	physical exam or physical education class
PERRL	pupils equal round and reactive to light
PHQ	Patient Health Questionnaire
PPE	pre-participation exam
PPS	peripheral pulmonary stenosis
QD or q	every day or just "every"
RDA	recommended daily allowance
ROM	range of motion
RV	rotavirus
S/NT/ND	soft, non-tender, non-distended
SDQ	Strengths and Difficulties Questionnaires
SIDS	sudden infant death syndrome
SMR	sexual maturity rating
SNAP	Supplemental Nutrition Assistance Program
SOAP	subjective, objective, assessment, and plan
STNR	symmetrical tonic neck reflex
STI	sexually transmitted infection
Tdap	tetanus, diphtheria, and acellular pertussis
THC	tetrahydrocannabinol (psychoactive component in marijuana)
TLR	tonic labyrinthine reflex
TM	tympanic membrane
UE	upper extremity
VAR	varicella
WCC	well-child check
WD/WN	well developed and well nourished
WHO	World Health Organization
WIC	Women, Infants, and Children